KU-687-039

TUBERCULOSIS

A SOURCEBOOK FOR NURSING PRACTICE

Felissa L. Cohen, RN, PhD, FAAN

Jerry D. Durham, RN, PhD, FAAN

Editors

CHESTER COLLEGE
ACC No.
0 0961323
CLASS No.
616.9950024 613
COH
LIBRARY

Springer Publishing Company

Copyright © 1995 by Springer Publishing Company, Inc.

All rights reserved

No part of this publication may be reproduced, stored in a retrieval system, or transmitted in any form or by any means, electronic, mechanical, photocopying, recording, or otherwise, without the prior permission of Springer Publishing Company, Inc.

Springer Publishing Company, Inc.
536 Broadway
New York, NY 10012-3955

Cover design by Tom Yabut

95 96 97 98 99 / 5 4 3 2 1

Library of Congress Cataloging-in-Publication Data

Tuberculosis : a sourcebook for nursing practice / Felissa L. Cohen, Jerry Durham, editors.
      p. cm.
      Includes bibliographical references and index.
      ISBN 0-8261-8720-X
      1. Tuberculosis—Nursing. 2. Tuberculosis. I. Cohen, Felissa L. II. Durham, Jerry D.
      [DNLM: 1. Tuberculosis—nursing. 2. Tuberculosis—prevention & control. WY 163 T885 1994]
RC311.8.T83   1994
616.9'95—dc20
DNLM/DLC
for Library of Congress   94–35452
                                      CIP

*To the special people in my life with much love:
my children—Peter, Heather, Neal, and Julie; my mother, Ruth Lashley;
and my special friend, Tony Oliver.*

Felissa Lashley Cohen

*To my brother, Benton Durham, for a lifetime of love, support,
and understanding.*

Jerry D. Durham

CONTENTS

Contributors

Janice A. Boutotte, RN, MS, CS, is Director of Epidemiology, Case Management, and Prevention Services at the Division of Tuberculosis Control, Massachusetts Department of Public Health, Jamaica Plain, Massachusetts. She is a TB consultant for the American Nurses Association (ANA) and represents ANA on the National Coalition for the Elimination of Tuberculosis. Ms. Boutotte is chairperson of the ANA's ad hoc TB Advisory Task Force.

Linda Edwards, RN, PhD, is Assistant Chair for Education at Rush University College of Nursing. She formerly was a practitioner/teacher in public health nursing at Rush University College of Nursing, Chicago, Illinois, and the School Health Coordinator for the Illinois Department of Public Health.

Sue Etkind, RN, MS, is Director, Division of Tuberculosis Control, Massachusetts Department of Public Health, Jamaica Plain, Massachusetts. Ms. Etkind has recently served as a member of the National Advisory Committee for the Elimination of Tuberculosis. She was the 1994 recipient of the Lillian Wald Service Award from the Public Health Nursing Section of the American Public Health Association.

Carol Davis Harriman, RN, MSN, MPH, is employed with the TB Control Program of the El Paso City/County Health and Environment District. She was formerly the director of the Health and Safety Department, Texas Tech University, Health Sciences Center, El Paso, Texas, and nurse consultant with the TB Control Program in the New Mexico Health Department.

Ann E. Kurth, RN, MSN, MPH, CNM, is Director of Clinical Data and Research, Division of Acquired Diseases, Indiana State Department of Health, Indianapolis, Indiana. She is a certified nurse midwife and has been involved with HIV disease research and education in both clinical and public health prevention settings.

Lorie Madsen, RN, BSN, CS, is a certified adult nurse practitioner and transtracheal oxygen coordinator for the mycobacterial disease service at National Jewish Center for Immunology and Respiratory Medicine (NJC) in Denver, Colorado. She is a member of the Mycobacterial Nurses Special Interest Group of the American Thoracic Society and is one of the speakers in the International TB course that is given at NJC.

Barbara McGinnis, RN, is TB nurse epidemiologist at Pine Street Inn, Boston, Massachusetts, for the City of Boston, Department of Health and Hospitals. She has received a humanitarian award from the Massachusetts Nurses Association and has been nationally recognized for her work with the homeless.

Elizabeth K. Peabody, RN, C MSN, is a certified adult nurse practitioner and pulmonary nurse practitioner at Richard L. Roudebush Veterans Administration Medical Center in Indianapolis, Indiana. She was formerly head nurse on a pulmonary unit and now follows patients with tuberculosis and other pulmonary diseases in an outpatient clinic.

Joan E. Otten, RN, BSN, is Director of the office of Tuberculosis Control, Jackson Memorial Medical Center, Miami, Florida. She is certified as a Healthcare Risk Manager by the American Institute of Medical Law.

Maureen Shekleton, RN, DNSc, is satellite site coordinator of the DuPage Community Clinic, Wheaton, Illinois, and is an adjunct faculty member at the University of Illinois at Chicago. She is past president of the Respiratory Nursing Society. Dr. Shekleton is the recipient of the 1994 Jessie M. Scott Award of the American Nurses association showing commitment to the integration of nursing research, education, and practice.

Helena Sibilano, RN, PhD, is a pulmonary clinical nurse specialist at the West Side Veterans Administration Hospital in Chicago, Illinois, and an adjunct faculty member at the University of Illinois College of Nursing. She is a member of the Tuberculosis Education Task Force of the American Nurses Association. Ms. Sibilano was the 1993 recipient of the Clinical Nurse Specialist Award from the Illinois Nurses Association.

Linda Singleton, RN, BS, MPH, is Director of Policy and Clinical Services, Division of Tuberculosis Control, Massachusetts Department of Public Health, Boston, Massachusetts. She has also been an infection control practitioner and home health agency administrator in Utah.

Esther Sumartojo, PhD, is a research psychologist, Clinical Research Branch, Division of Tuberculosis Elimination, National Center for Prevention Services, Centers for Disease Control and Prevention, Atlanta, Georgia. Dr. Sumartojo is responsible for developing a research agenda for behavioral studies related to TB.

Maria A. Tricarico, RN, MA, CNAA, is Director of Patient Care Services at Lemuel Shattuck Hospital in Boston, Massachusetts. She collaborated on and administered the development of a model inpatient TB treatment unit at Lemuel Shattuck Hospital with the TB Division of the Massachusetts Department of Public Health.

PREFACE

"Too late, too late. Well, I got the TB and the TB's all in my bones, in my bones. . . ."[1]

Immortalized both in music and literature, tuberculosis (TB) has affected humans since 5000 BC and has been widely feared.

" . . . T.B.'s is killin' me . . . T.B.'s is killin' me. Got the tuberculosis, consumption is killin' me . . . Well, you see I got the TB—now I'm dead and gone."

Variously known as "consumption," "white death," "white plague," and " . . . the Captain of All These Men of Death," a diagnosis of TB before the 1940s was often a death sentence.

" . . . I'm on my way to Denver. God knows I can't hesitate. . . ."

---

[1]Song lyrics from "TB Blues" as performed by Champion Jack Dupree. *Blues from the Gutter*, Atlanta Recording Corp., 1992.

Therapeutic approaches such as fresh air, particularly mountain air, sunshine, skilled nursing care, and rest were widely advocated but not available to all. The discovery of streptomycin, para aminosalicylic acid, and isoniazid, and their concomitant use of treat TB ushered in a new era of treatment. As effective treatment and prevention programs led to the control of TB, particularly in the developed countries, complacency set in. Tuberculosis sanitoriums that had developed specifically for the quarantine of TB patients began to be phased out and were closed in this country by the mid- to late-1960s.

> *" . . . Well, the TB is all right to have, but your friends treat you so low down, so low down . . . Don't ask them no favors; they'll stop comin' round, comin' round."*

These song lyrics express the stigmatization and isolation that was often felt by those who were quarantined and separated from their families and friends. Today, those affected by illnesses such as TB and HIV disease fear disclosing their illness or burdening others with requests for help and support.

Nurses caring for persons with TB and their families carry a special responsibility to model ethical, compassionate, nonjudgmental care and to dispel harmful myths that may exist about TB among their colleagues, clients, and the general public. The "diseases" of ignorance and prejudice can inflict as much damage on those with TB as can the causative bacterium.

Until health officials began sounding warnings in the mid-1980s, when cases of TB began to increase in the United States, TB had largely slipped from public view and awareness in the United States. Conditions that always nurtured TB development—poverty, poor nutrition, crowding, and unsanitary living conditions—became evident again in this country. Combined with substance use, homelessness, a high prevalence of populations with latent tuberculous infection, and the emergence of the HIV epidemic, TB found new fertile ground in which to grow. Added to this were the decline of funding for TB programs, decreased TB-related research, the more passive and complacent approach to the long-term TB therapy, difficulties in maintaining contact with patients to promote adherence, and the eventual emergence of multidrug-resistant TB (MDR-TB) strains.

In other parts of the world, TB has continued to exact a terrible toll. Tuberculosis remains the single greatest cause of death from infectious disease, representing almost one-fifth of adult deaths in developing countries. Each year eight million new cases are reported, and three million persons perish from TB.

This nation's health-care providers and educators seem now to have awakened to the reality that Americans are citizens of TB's "global village." Content regarding prevention, assessment, diagnosis, and treatment of TB has begun receiving new emphasis in nursing and medical curricula. Practitioners are now increasingly alert to the possibility of TB in patients, particularly those from groups considered as being at greater risk of infection than the general population. Funding for research and demonstration projects, particularly for populations at higher risk of TB and/or nonadherence to therapeutic regimens, has increased significantly. Concerns about the underlying social conditions that give rise to TB have focused new attention on the decline of the public health infrastructure in this nation. Tuberculosis's resurgence has also refocused attention on the effectiveness of primary prevention and early intervention in controlling disease at an important time juncture in the current national debate on health-care reform.

Few books emphasizing TB with a nursing focus have been written in recent times. The spectrum of TB-related nursing activities is wide. This book's primary purpose is to provide nurses and other health-care professionals with the knowledge to allow them to provide effective care for those with or at risk of acquiring TB. Today's TB nurse specialists must keep abreast of emerging developments in the biomedical and social sciences that can affect the treatment plan. Furthermore, nurses should advocate for the appropriate intervention to prevent transmission of communicable and infectious diseases in individual and congregate settings such as hospitals, institutions, and schools.

Finally, nurses should take heed and apply an important lesson of the HIV epidemic: Allowing fear and hysteria to shape health care and public policy is not only detrimental for person with TB but serves to distract us from a duty to care. As this nation's largest group of health-care practitioners, nurses have a duty to model our profession's long-standing commitment to provide effective and compassionate care for persons with TB in an environment that promotes safe practice. This book provides readers with the necessary knowledge base to meet this professional right and obligation.

FELISSA LASHLEY COHEN
JERRY D. DURHAM

PART I
Background

TUBERCULOSIS: AN INTRODUCTION

Felissa L. Cohen and Jerry D. Durham

It is a common misconception that infectious diseases have been virtually eradicated. Worldwide, however, infectious diseases are still the leading cause of death, and tuberculosis (TB) is the leading cause of death among the infectious diseases. In the United States, the incidence of TB had been generally declining until 1986 when an increase in cases was seen (Bloom & Murray, 1992). HIV infection/AIDS is one of the major factors contributing to that rise, but social, economic, and political factors have also played a role. The resurgence of TB and the appearance of multidrug-resistant TB have caused new concern and focus on this disease. This chapter provides brief background information about TB and places the rise in TB cases in a historical context.

WHAT IS TUBERCULOSIS?

Tuberculosis (TB) may be broadly defined as a chronic, communicable, bacterial disease caused by tubercle bacilli. Tubercle bacilli include several members of the bacterial genus *Mycobacterium* that are sometimes

TABLE 1.1   Some Factors Influencing the Occurrence of Tuberculous Infection

Factors Relating to the Host

Nutritional status
Stress
Genetic predisposition and other innate characteristics
Immune competence
Nature and volume of respiratory secretions
Presence of other diseases

Factors Relating to the Organism

Virulence of strain
Concentration of *M. tuberculosis* in droplet nuclei
Size and number of aerosolized droplets

Factors Relating to the Environment

Crowding
Unclean living conditions
Fresh air ventilation
Indoor air volume

Other

Contact with source patient
　Length of time
　Duration
　Closeness
Source patient characteristics
　Symptoms
　Cavitary or noncavitary disease
　Site of TB
　TB medication status—type and length of time
　Positive or negative sputum smear

referred to as the "tuberculosis complex." In the United States, *Mycobacterium tuberculosis* is the most important and common cause of TB. *M. tuberculosis* is a nonmotile, nonspore forming, rod-shaped bacillus that has no capsule and does not produce toxin. It is commonly known as "acid fast" because of certain characteristics regarding the staining used in microbiology. The tubercle bacillus is hardy, and it can remain dormant for long periods under adverse conditions. It is, however, an obligate aerobe whose growth is dependent on adequate oxygen tension. This need for adequate oxygen is a major reason for its preference for oxygen-rich tissue such as the lung. When deprived of oxygen, its growth is slowed or stopped (Grosset, 1993; Joklik, Willett, Amos, & Wilfert, 1992; MacGregor, 1993; Moulding, 1994).

TRANSMISSION

The major route of TB transmission is from person to person through the inhalation of airborne particles that contain *M. tuberculosis*. These particles are referred to as droplet nuclei. They are produced when a person with infectious TB of the lungs or larynx forcefully exhales. Forced expiratory maneuvers that generate these aerosolized droplet nuclei include coughing, sneezing, singing, yelling, and loud talking. These small droplet nuclei can remain suspended in the air. Persons sharing the same air space as a person with active tuberculosis can then inhale the droplets. Although the majority of cases of TB in the United States are transmitted through inhalation, transmission can also occur through ingestion of contaminated food or drink or through direct inoculation (Centers for Disease Control and Prevention, 1993; Frampton, 1992; Hutton, Stead, Cauthen, Bloch, & Ewing, 1990; Kramer, Sasse, Simms, & Leedom, 1993; Nardell, 1993). Various factors influence whether or not tuberculous infection occurs in a person exposed to *M. tuberculosis*. These include factors relating to the organism, host, environment, and their interaction. These are shown in Table 1.1. The risk of acquiring tuberculous infection increases with the length of time the susceptible person shares the air space with the person who has active tuberculosis.

The most common site for tuberculosis is pulmonary, and more than 80% of cases occur in the lung. TB can also occur in extrapulmonary sites, particularly where oxygen-rich tissue is present. Common extrapulmonary sites include the larynx, lymph nodes, kidney, bone, and brain. Extrapulmonary TB, with or without pulmonary TB, is frequently found in persons with HIV-disease (Centers for Disease and Prevention, 1993; Haas & Des Prez, 1994; Slutsker, Castro, Ward, & Dooley, 1993).

TUBERCULOUS INFECTION AND TUBERCULOSIS

It is important to understand the difference between tuberculous infection and tuberculosis. Tuberculous infection may be present with or without disease (tuberculosis). Individuals who have living tubercle bacilli present without clinically active disease are considered to have tuberculous infection. These individuals

- have tubercle bacilli in their body;
- are usually infected for life;
- usually have a positive reaction to the tuberculin skin test;
- are not infectious to others;
- usually have a negative chest radiograph;
- usually do not have clinical symptoms of tuberculosis;
- usually have negative sputum cultures and smears for tubercle bacilli;
- may be at risk for contracting clinical disease, especially if their immune system becomes compromised; and
- may be candidates for preventive therapy (Centers for Disease Control and Prevention, 1993.)

The vast majority (about 90%) of people in the United States who acquire tuberculous infection do not develop tuberculosis because their immune system activity successfully contains the tubercle bacilli, although the precise mechanism has not been completely elucidated (Rook, 1994). The risk for a person with tuberculous infection in the United States to develop tuberculosis is about 5% in the first year or 2 after infection and another 5% during their lifetime (Centers for Disease Control and Prevention, 1993; Dunlap & Briles, 1993).

Individuals who have active pulmonary tuberculosis

- are infected with *M. tuberculosis*;
- usually have a positive reaction to the tuberculin skin test;
- usually have clinical symptoms (although these may be nonspecific);
- usually have positive sputum smears and/or cultures for tubercle bacilli before therapy; and
- may be infectious to others before treatment is effective (Centers for Disease Control and Prevention, 1993).

SCREENING, DETECTION, AND DIAGNOSIS OF TUBERCULOSIS

Screening programs have long been a mainstay of the public health TB prevention programs. Aims include identifying those with tuberculous infection who could benefit from preventive therapy and finding those with tuberculosis who need treatment. The usual screening programs employ tuberculin skin tests, such as the Mantoux test, for detection of tuberculous infection and may also use chest radiography. Guidelines for interpreting the Mantoux test depend upon risk factors for the person being tested that may be personal or related to employment or residence (American Thoracic Society, 1992). These are discussed in Chapter 8. Persons identified as reactive on the Mantoux test need appropriate further diagnostic testing, and if indicated, preventive therapy or medical treatment. These are discussed in Chapters 4 and 5.

SYMPTOMS OF TUBERCULOSIS

Tuberculosis may present clinically in a variety of ways and may vary according to the site of the disease. The most common presentation of pulmonary TB is an insidious one with the gradual development of vague symptoms. Common symptoms include

- cough, usually productive, occasionally with blood-streaked sputum
- fatigue or malaise
- anorexia
- weight loss
- low grade fever, often occurring in the afternoon, may be intermittent
- sweating and/or chills at night
- dull, aching chest pain or tightness (MacGregor, 1993; Schluger & Rom, 1994).

All of the above symptoms may not be present, and the severity of a particular symptom may be variable. Diagnosis of TB on the basis of symptoms alone is difficult. In the elderly, for example, symptoms may be subtle (Couser & Glassroth, 1993). In those with HIV-infection, symptoms can be attributed to other compounding illnesses or to HIV-disease itself, or the presentation may be atypical. Those persons with HIV-infection should be evaluated for TB periodically (DiFerdinando, Glassroth, Hecht, & Stover, 1993). In those with HIV-infection, TB occurs most frequently through reactivation of a latent tuberculous infection but can also occur through the acquisition of primary progressive disease (Barnes, Le, & Davidson, 1993; Centers for Disease Control and Prevention, 1993). In extrapulmonary TB the symptoms manifested will be related to the affected organ system. Nonspecific symptoms may also be seen. Clinicians must be alert to the possibility of TB when a patient exhibits even a few of the classic symptoms or is at particular risk for the development of TB and implement the appropriate diagnostic procedures (Schluger, & Rom, 1994).

TREATMENT

The mainstay of treatment for pulmonary TB has been drug therapy. Several drugs have been used traditionally, and new ones have been added. Decision making for an optimum drug treatment regimen includes evaluation for the risk that multidrug-resistant TB (MDR-TB) may be present and whether or not the person with TB is coinfected with HIV. Treatment plans, issues, and monitoring are discussed in Chapters 5 and 6. Adherence over a long period of medication administration has been shown to be a major issue in therapeutic success. Directly observed therapy is one approach to maximizing adherence. Adherence is discussed in Chapter 7, and other approaches to therapy in Chapters 10, 12, and 13.

A BRIEF HISTORY OF PULMONARY TUBERCULOSIS

In 1882, Robert Koch announced that tuberculosis was caused by *Mycobacterium tuberculosis*, the tubercle bacilli. This discovery ultimately led to ways of decreasing transmission and effective treatment modalities. Prior to Koch's discovery, TB was believed to be constitutional, a form of tumor or abnormal gland (Bloom & Murray, 1992). In the 1870s and 1880s, scientists generally held that TB resulted from hereditary predisposition, juxtaposed with a bad environment and/or improper living (Bates, 1992).

   Tuberculosis (TB) is an ancient disease. Physical evidence from Egyptian mummies and Stone Age skeletons suggests that TB has existed in humans since antiquity (Bloom and Murray, 1992; Joklik, et al. 1992; Zimmerman, 1979). TB was epidemic in Europe in the 18th and 19th centuries when vast numbers of people died from it. TB has been variously called, "consumption," "phthisis," "the white death," "the white plague," and "captain of all these men of death." Until the 20th century, TB was the most important cause of death among adults (Bloom et al. Murray, 1992; Keers, 1978; Meyer, 1991). Even today TB remains the leading cause of death among infectious diseases worldwide (Bloom et al., 1992).

   Koch's discovery of the cause of TB, unfortunately, did not result in its cure, although his premature announcement in 1890 that he had discovered a substance to prevent the development of tubercle bacilli in humans created a sensation (Leibowitz, 1993). Even before Koch's discovery, the belief that sunlight, healthful food, and fresh air could fight tuberculosis took hold (Earnest & Sbarbaro, 1993). Hermann Brehmer established the first sanatorium in 1854 in Europe with the theory that altitude and exercise could cure TB (Bloom et al., 1993). In the belief that the aroma of spruce or pine trees was therapeutic, sanatoriums were established in mountainous areas, particularly in New York State (e.g., The Ray Brook State Tuberculosis Hospital, the Sunmount Veterans Administration Hospital, and the Will Rogers Sanatorium), Colorado, and North Carolina (especially near Asheville) (Meyer, 1991). Unprecedented health campaigns (e.g., the Easter Seal Campaign) against TB swept the nation in the first half of the 20th century.

> America banned together to fight the scourge. Parents were urged to leave windows open to expel bad air and protect their children; public schools initiated hygiene classes; posters and flyers covered walls and kiosks across the country, trumpeting measures thought to combat the disease. . . .Tuberculosis acquired a moral dimension that eerily foreshadowed some of the more extreme responses to AIDS; if the disease arose from unhealthy habits, it followed logically that to continue to live in such conditions—to dwell in crowded tenements, to persist in a life of poverty—was irresponsible and immoral, a threat to clean-living citizens everywhere (Earnest et al., 1993, p.16).

Bates (1992) argues that the building of institutions for treatment of consumptives sprang from three main goals: (1) an institution could "correct the moral decay of an urban society and . . . save the souls of the helplessly ill" (p.330); (2) segregation could prevent the spread of disease to others; and (3) treatment in an institution could effect cure, thus returning a patient to a productive life. A fourth goal of institutions, never fully realized, was linking care to eradication of TB through research. During the era of institutionalization of TB patients, home care was largely unsuccessful as a strategy to treat and prevent TB (Bates, 1992). During this period, however, African-Americans were largely cared for in the home since institutional care was either unavailable to them or, if available, was substandard (Bates, 1992).

Institutionalized patients were expected to yield to medical authority in return for care and treatment. As is also seen today, care providers often overestimated their patients' ability or willingness to adhere to therapy or change behaviors. It was not uncommon for some to leave the sanatorium while still infectious (Bates, 1992).

The role of nurses in the battle against TB in the late 19th and early 20th centuries was significant and has been described by LaMotte (1985) and Bates (1992). It is noteworthy that some of the earliest nurses themselves had been afflicted with TB (Bates, 1992). Today, nurses and other health care providers are also at risk for acquiring tuberculous infection in the occupational setting. LaMotte's book, first published in 1915, contains content ranging from the nurse's training and visiting instructions to inspection of the house and care of the family. Visiting nurse societies of the late 19th and early 20th centuries were formed to help the poor, and TB patients were among those they served.

In the decades before the introduction of chemotherapy, the armamentaria in the battle against TB had been highly unpredictable in bringing about a cure. In addition to segregation of TB patients (and sometimes their families), chaulmoogra oil (a tree derivative once used to treat leprosy) and various chemicals, dyes, metal salts, and antibiotics (e.g., sulfonamides and penicillin) were tried. Surgical intervention, called "collapse therapy" (i.e., therapeutic or artificial pneumothorax), involved the injection of air into the pleural space to effect lung "collapse," thus allowing the infected lung to rest. If this intervention was unsuccessful, thoracoplasty or phrenic crush might also be tried to decrease the lung's mobility and/or effect cavity closure. Although these procedures were not without complications (e.g., infection, hemoptysis, sudden death) some patients improved or recovered from their disease (Bates, 1992; Meyer, 1991). Thoracoplasty was the most successful of the surgical interventions prior to the introduction of chemotherapy and was reported to have returned thousands of patients to a normal life (Meyer, 1991).

Treatment of TB prior to the introduction of chemotherapy was largely aimed at its early diagnosis. By the late 1930s diagnosis could be established in those believed to be infected through tuberculin skin tests and radiographs (Bates, 1992). Once diagnosed, the patient's family members could be examined and the patient could be offered treatment, often in a sanatorium. Those with the means could travel to better climates for treatment in private sanatoriums. From 1900 to 1940, care of TB patients gradually shifted from homes to institutions, largely government supported. During this period, few African-Americans entered sanitoriums, even the public ones, because the facilities were segregated. Because of the Depression, however, most private sanatoriums had disappeared by the 1930s (Bates, 1992).

Following the introduction of chemotherapy, the care of TB patients began to shift from sanatoriums to general hospitals, hastened by a recommendation by the American College of Chest Physicians (1972). By 1973, only 17 states had TB sanatoriums, and by 1981 most of these states had also begun to use general hospitals for TB treatment (Rieder, 1989). The sanatoriums had become largely obsolete with the advent of short hospitalizations and ambulatory treatment. Over time, most of these sanatoriums were demolished or converted to other uses.

The discovery of drugs to treat TB effectively held the potential for a cure and marked dramatic changes in care delivery. Streptomycin was discovered in 1943 by Selman Waksman (Earnest & Sbarbaro, 1993), followed by 11 more drugs by 1967, although only two, isoniazid and rifampin, were considered first-line drugs. Drug treatment allowed for most persons with active TB to be cured within a few months and to return to normal lives within a few weeks after chemotherapy began. Thus, the major challenges in TB treatment then, as today, included prevention activities, early identification of infected individuals, and implementation of interventions to ensure their adherence to treatment.

Although the HIV/AIDS epidemic has more recently highlighted the damaging elements of fear on society, fear also played an important role in the battle against TB in the early 20th century during the anti-TB campaigns. Growing concerns about TB in the early 20th century fed xenophobia and a nativism movement, resulting in restrictive immigration laws, possibly aimed at the "germs" of socialism and anarchism (Rothman, 1992). The association of TB and poverty also led to the labeling of persons with TB as "one lungers." Fear of TB during this era even had a name: phthistiophobia (Rothman, 1992).

The role of fear in the social history of TB has been summarized by Bates.

> Physicians and other propagandists used fear of infection to encourage hygienic habits, promote legislation, build institutions, and persuade patients to enter them and accept proper discipline. Campaigners argued that the public was thus protecting itself and that patients were saving themselves from death and protecting their families. . . . Men and women, stigmatized by the diagnosis, found their friends avoiding them and had more than the usual problems in finding jobs. . . . When campaigners portrayed the tuberculous poor and tuberculous blacks as dangerous to the rest of society, they were often trying to create a system of care for them. If people had not been made to feel anxious, they might have responded much less generously." (pp.333-334).

Gradually, as the TB became more treatable, fear of those who were infected began to decline. However, the fears and subsequent behaviors demonstrated by society in this and prior centuries when faced with the threat of death from communicable diseases resurfaced in the era of AIDS.

CONCLUSION

Even though TB has claimed millions of lives worldwide in the 20th century, once a cure was discovered, most Americans no longer considered TB a threat. Its resurgence, at a time of growing concern about contagion, largely related to the HIV epidemic, surprised many, including health care providers, who had incorrectly assumed that TB was all but eradicated or was found only among marginal groups. This lack of awareness and complacency provided fertile grounds for TB to grow. Patients' nonadherence to therapy, always a challenge to health care providers, has taken on new significance in the present epidemic, particularly among the poor and those with HIV infection. Primary challenges to health care providers, particularly in the public health sector, include preventing the spread of TB through effective screening, case finding and diagnosis, and limiting the impact of TB among infected persons through careful monitoring and treatment approaches.

Nurses have historically played important roles in the care and treatment of persons with TB, including case finding, home care, and institutional care. Administering medications, providing comfort measures, working with families, referring patients to sources of assistance, monitoring patients' adherence to treatment plans, and maintaining a safe environment are TB-related nursing activities, which have been chronicled from the inception of modern nursing until today. Nurses today are augmenting these roles with activities in such areas as research, public policy, education, and health services administration.

REFERENCES

American College of Chest Physicians. (1972). Report of the Committee on Tuberculosis: Utilization of general hospitals in the treatment of tuberculosis. *Chest, 61,* 405.

American Thoracic Society. (1992). Control of tuberculosis in the United States. *American Review of Respiratory Disease, 146,* 1623–1633.

Barnes, P.F., Le, H.Q., & Davidson, P.T. (1993). Tuberculosis in patients with HIV infection. *Medical Clinics of North America, 77(6),* 1369–1390.

Bates, B. (1992). Bargaining for life: A social history of tuberculosis, 1876–1938. Philadelphia: University of Pennsylvania.

Bloom, B. & Murray, C. (1992). Tuberculosis: Commentary on a reemergent killer. *Science, 257,* 1055–1063.

Centers for Disease Control and Prevention. (1993). *TB/HIV—the connection:*

*what health care workers should know.*Atlanta: Centers for Disease Control and Prevention.

Couser, J. I., Jr. & Glassroth, J. (1993). Tuberculosis. An epidemic in older adults. *Clinics in Chest Medicine,14*(3),491–499.

DiFernando, G.T., Jr., Glassroth, J., Hecht, F.M., & Stover, D.E. (1993). TB and HIV: A deadly synergy. *Patient Care, 27(14)*, 92–114.

Dunlap, N.E., & Briles, D.E. (1993). Immunology of tuberculosis. *Medical Clinics of North America,77*, 1235–1251.

Earnest, M., & Sbarbaro, J. (1993). A plague returns. *The Sciences, 33* (5), 14–19.

Frampton, M.W. (1992). An outbreak of tuberculosis among hospital personnel caring for a patient with a skin ulcer. *Annals of Internal Medicine, 117*, 312–313.

Grosset, J.H. (1993). Bacteriology of tuberculosis. *Lung Biology in Health and Disease, 66*, 49–79.

Haas, D.W., & Des Pres, R.M. (1994). Tuberculosis and acquired immunodeficiency syndrome: A historical perspective on recent developments. *American Journal of Medicine, 96*, 439–450.

Hutton, M.D., Stead, W.W., Cauthen, G.M., Bloch, A.B., & Ewing, W.M. (1990). Nosocomial transmission of tuberculosis associated with a draining abscess. *Journal of Infectious Diseases, 161*, 286–295.

Joklik, W.K., Willett, H.P., Amos, D.B., & Wilfert, C.M. (1992). *Zinsser microbiolgy.* (20th ed.), Norwalk, CT: Appleton & Lange.

Keers, R. (1978). Pulmonary tuberculosis: A journey down the centuries. London: Bailliere Tindall.

Kramer, F., Sasse, S.A., Simms, J.C., & Leedom, J.M. (1993). Primary cutaneous tuberculosis after a needlestick injury from a patient with AIDS and undiagnosed tuberculosis. *Annals of Internal Medicine, 119*, 594–595.

LaMotte, E. (1985). The tuberculosis nurse. NY: Garland.

Leibowitz, D. (1993). Scientific failure in an age of optimism: Public reaction to Robert Koch's tuberculin cure. *New York State Journal of Medicine, 93*, 41–48.

MacGregor, R. R. (1993). Tuberculosis: From history to current management. *Seminars in Roentgenology, XXVIII (2)*, 101–108.

Meyer, J. (1991). Tuberculosis, the Adirondacks, and the coming of age of thoracic surgery. *Annals of Thoracic Surgery, 52*, 881–885.

Moulding, T. (1994). Pathophysiology and immunology: Clinical aspects. In D. Schlossberg (Ed)., *Tuberculosis* (3rd ed.). (pp. 41–50). New York: Springer-Verlag.

Nardell, E. A. (1993). Pathogenesis of tuberculosis. *Lung Biology in Health and Disease, 66*, 103–122. Reider, H. (1989). Tuberculosis among American indians of the contiguous United States. *Public Health Reports, 104*, 653–657.

Rook, G.A. (1994). Macrophages and *Mycobacterium tuberculosis*: The key to pathogenesis. In B.S. Zwilling & T.K. Eisenstein (Eds). *Macrophage-pathogen interactions*, (pp. 249–261). New York: Marcel Dekker, Inc.

Rothman, S. (1992). The sanitorium experience: Myths and realities. In *United*

Hospital Fund, The tuberculosis revival: Individual rights and societal obligations in a time of AIDS (pp. 67–73). NY: Author.

Schluger, N.W., & Rom, W.N. (1994). Current approaches to the diagnosis of active pulmonary tuberculosis. *American Journal of Respiratory and Critical Care Medicine, 149*, 264–267.

Slutsker, L., Castro, K. G., Ward, J. W., & Dooley, S. W., Jr. (1993). Epidemiology of extrapulmonary tuberculosis among persons with AIDS in the United States. *Clinical Infectious Diseases, 16*, 513–518.

Zimmerman, M. (1979). Pulmonary and osseous tuberculosis in an Egyptian mummy. *Bulletin of the New York Academy of Medicine, 55*, 604–608.

2

THE ETIOLOGY, TRANSMISSION, AND PATHOGENESIS OF TUBERCULOSIS

Maureen Shekleton

The ability to devise effective strategies for disease control and to evaluate an exposed person's risk of becoming infected with tuberculosis depend on the clinician's understanding of the factors that govern transmission of the disease as well as its sequence of development. This chapter discusses the etiology, microbiology, and pathogenesis of tuberculosis, and factors that determine disease development and progression. The role of infection with the human immunodeficiency virus (HIV) is described, since it is currently recognized as being the most important acquired risk factor for developing tuberculosis (Murray, 1989).

ETIOLOGY

Robert Koch announced his discovery of the cause of tuberculosis in 1882—*Mycobacterium tuberculosis*, the tubercle bacillus. However, effective drug therapy was not available until the 1940s. Today, tubercle bacilli include several members of the genus *Mycobacterium*, sometimes referred to as "the tuberculosis complex," including *Mycobacterium tuberculosis, M. bovis, M. africanum*, and rarely, *M. microti* (Grosset, 1993; Witebsky & Conville, 1993). Of these, *M. tuberculosis* is the most common and important in this country. *M. bovis* is most often transmitted through unpasturized milk, and *M. africanum* is essentially confined to northwest Africa; therefore, both have little importance in this country (Comstock & Cauthen, 1993). In this book, discussion will be largely confined to *M. tuberculosis*.

MICROBIOLOGY

M. tuberculosis is a nonmotile, nonspore forming, rod-shaped bacillus that ranges in size from 0.2 to 0.6 microns in width and 1 to 5 microns in length, has no capsule, and does not produce toxin. It is known as "acid-fast" because the lipid in its cell wall makes it resistant to the usual Gram stain, and resistant to decolorization with acid-alcohol. Thus, staining approaches of Ziehl-Neelsen and Kinyoun techniques are used to visualize it under the microscope, making the bacilli appear as red-staining rods (Joklik, Willett, Amos, & Wilfert, 1992; MacGregor, 1993). Fluorescent staining, such as with auramine or auramine-rhodamine, is also used with the accompanying microscopy (MacGregor, 1993). Because the cell wall is high in lipid content, mycobacteria are resistant to chemical injury from certain chemical agents normally used in disinfection such as sodium hydroxide and detergents. It is sensitive to formaldehyde and glutaraldehyde. It can stay viable for weeks at 4° and for several years at -70°. *M. tuberculosis* can survive for long periods under adverse conditions, and its hardiness allows it to remain dormant and survive to cause disease under favorable conditions years after primary infection has occurred. It is however, susceptible to ultraviolet radiation, heat, and alcohol (Sherris, 1990).

    M. tuberculosis has a slow rate of growth (dividing every 18 to 24 hours or longer as opposed to *Escherichia coli* which divides in less than 1 hour) and needs enriched culture media in order to grow in the laboratory. Another important characteristic of *M. tuberculosis* is that it is an obligate aerobe whose growth is dependent on adequate oxygen tension. When deprived of oxygen, its multipication is slowed or stopped (Dunlap & Briles, 1993; Grosset, 1993; Joklik et al., 1992; MacGregor, 1993; Moulding, 1994). Thus, it can multiply rapidly in tuberculous lung cavities but much more slowly in caseous lung foci (necrotic areas that are cheeselike in consistency) where the oxygen tension is lower. Lung tissue that is high in oxygen is the most common target, but other tissue rich in oxygen such as the kidneys, vertebral bodies, lymph nodes, meningeal areas close to the subarachnoid space, and the epiphyseal areas (growing ends) of the long bones are also commonly affected (Mandell, Douglas & Bennett, 1990).

Like other microorganisms, tubercle bacilli can mutate, affecting such characteristics as virulence, biochemical characteristics, appearance of cultured colonies, and drug sensitivity. The latter is of great importance in regard to therapy. In the past, it has been most typical for mutation for drug resistance to be for one given drug, and to be sensitive to other agents, allowing clinicians to treat patients effectively with drug combinations. The evolution of multidrug-resistant strains of mycobacteria through mutation has therefore initiated many therapeutic problems that are discussed in Chapters 3 and 5.

TRANSMISSION

Transmission of infection involves the transfer of M. tuberculosis from a source to a new host. The most important route of transmission is through inhalation; transmission rarely occurs through ingestion of contaminated food or drink or through direct inoculation (Kramer, Sasse, Simms, & Leedom, 1993; Murray and Mills, 1990; Nardell, 1993). Most commonly, the tubercle bacillus is inhaled into the lungs via aerosolized airborne particles called droplet nuclei. Viable M. tuberculosis organisms are expelled from the lungs of individuals with pulmonary tuberculosis when they generate aerosolized particles through forced expiratory maneuvers such as coughing, sneezing, yelling, singing, and loud talking. All of these actions create a sudden acceleration of air that can move and disrupt the respiratory secretions creating aerosolized droplets. Once airborne, the water content of the aerosolized secretions rapidly evaporates leaving behind the droplet nucleus, a residue of solid matter containing the tubercle bacillus (Hopewell, 1988; Moulding, 1983; Nardell, 1990).

Factors that affect the likelihood of transmission of M. tuberculosis from an infected person to a new host include the characteristics of the aerosolized droplets that are generated, the environmental conditions to which the droplet nuclei are exposed, and the circumstances under which contact with the new host occur (Hopewell, 1988; Murray, 1989). Characteristics of the aerosolized droplets that affect transmission include their size, number, and the bacilli concentration. The smaller the droplet size, the greater the number of droplets, and the higher the concentration of bacilli conveyed in droplets, the more likely it is that transmission will occur.

Size of the droplet is important because only the smallest airborne particles (1–5 microns) can be inhaled into the alveolus. Particles of 10 microns in diameter or larger are filtered in the nose, and particles between 5-10 microns are cleared by the mucociliary clearance system. The smaller the size (diameter) of the particle, the deeper it is able to penetrate into the respiratory system, thus reaching the alveolar surface where infection can be established. As compared to larger particles that tend to settle out of the air and deposit on surfaces, the smaller droplets continue to remain suspended within the air and, as airborne particles, can be inhaled over longer periods of time, also increasing the likelihood of transmission (Edwards & Kirkpatrick, 1986; Hopewell, 1988; Hopewell, 1993; Moulding, 1983; Reynolds, 1987).

The size and number of droplets are determined by the nature and volume of the respiratory tract secretions and the frequency of their expulsion into the atmosphere. Thin, watery respiratory secretions are more easily broken up into small droplets than thick mucus secretions. The larger the volume of the respiratory tract secretions, the greater the number of droplets that can be generated. The volume of droplets being generated will also be increased as the frequency of coughing or other forced expiratory maneuvers increases (Clancy, 1990; Hopewell, 1988). It is estimated that one cough can release about 3,000 droplet nuclei, and that less than 10 tubercle bacilli can initiate infection (Sherris, 1990).

In persons with pulmonary tubercular lesions, the bacilli concentration will reflect the extent and type of lung pathology that is present. Cavitary lung lesions have much larger bacillary populations than solid, nodular lesions (Moulding, 1983; Hopewell, 1988). With a larger bacillary population existing in the lung tissue, it is more likely that greater numbers of bacilli will escape with each forced expiratory maneuver, thus increasing the likelihood that transmission will occur.

Once the organisms are expelled from the lungs of an infected person, the chances of transmission are lessened if the concentration of viable *M. tuberculosis* in the air can be reduced. The environment to which the organisms are exposed will determine their viability. The concentration of viable organisms in the air can be reduced by removing them through effective air filtration or killing them with ultraviolet radiation. Concentration is obviously less when droplets are distributed throughout large volumes of outside air.

The circumstances of the contact between the source case and the new host will also affect transmission. The more prolonged and intense the exposure, the greater the likelihood that transmission will occur (Murray, 1989). Lengthy and close contact most often occurs between family members or individuals living in overcrowded housing conditions. Examples of situations in which unintentional close contact or overcrowding might occur include temporary living shelters, jails, long-term care facilities, submarines, and low-income housing developments. The condition of a person living in poverty is often characterized by transient and/or overcrowded housing as well as malnutrition and poor hygiene, the latter being host factors that affect the pathogenesis of the disease process.

In summary, not everyone who inhales tubercle bacilli becomes infected. Other factors determine whether or not infection occurs. Small droplet nuclei that contain viable tubercle bacilli capable of causing infection must reach the peripheral lung of a susceptible individual. Factors influencing this include factors related to the host's ability to mount an adequate defense, bacterial characteristics such as the number and the virulence of the strain, and environmental conditions. The concentration of droplet nuclei in an area is increased when more are generated, when the indoor air volume is small, and when fresh air ventilation is low (Nardell, 1990). Thus, procedures that promote coughing, such as fiberoptic bronchoscopy or aerosolized pentamidine treatment (used in the treatment of *Pneumocystis carinii* pneumonia, most often seen in persons with HIV-disease), can release more droplet nuclei into the air.

Can a Person Catch TB From Riding Public Transportation? The answer to that question is, "It depends." As discussed above, key elements are the ventilation, the volume of air, the presence of someone with active TB, the closeness and duration of contact with that person, the presence of droplet nuclei, the size and concentration of droplet nuclei, the host's ability to mount a defense against the tubercle bacilli including past exposure to them, presence of other disease processes, innate characteristics of the host, the competency of the immune system, and virulence of the particular strain of *M. tuberculosis*. Factors that determine whether or not infection occurs are discussed in the next section.

PATHOGENESIS

It is important to understand the difference between tuberculous infection and tuberculosis. Tuberculous infection may be present with or without disease (tuberculosis). Persons who have living tubercle bacilli present without clinically active disease are considered to have tuberculous infection. Such individuals usually have a positive tuberculin skin test but do not have symptoms of tuberculosis and have negative bacteriologic studies. They are not infectious to others. Those individuals with tuberculous infection are at risk of contracting clinical disease, particularly if their immune system becomes impaired. Such a conversion may not take place for years, if at all. Persons who have tuberculosis are those who are not only infected with *M. tuberculosis*, usually having a positive tuberculin skin test, but who have clinically active disease usually with symptoms (although sometimes these are nonspecific) and who are infectious to others (American Thoracic Society, 1992; Centers for Disease Control, 1990).

The pathogenesis of tuberculosis occurs in two phases: (1) the initial (primary) infection with tubercle bacilli and (2) the subsequent development of tuberculosis (Hopewell, 1988). The pathogenesis of tuberculosis depends on a number of factors such as the host's innate body defenses, nutritional status, age and, possibly, the dose of bacteria implanted in the lungs (inoculum effect).

The droplet nuclei that are inhaled and are small enough to reach and implant on the alveolar surface usually contain only a few tubercle bacilli. If this is the person's first encounter with TB, alveolar macrophages that normally scavenge the alveolar surface ingest the tubercle bacilli and can kill or remove them. This nonimmunologic response can be effective in preventing infection if relatively few bacilli are implanted on the alveolar surface. Other factors influencing outcome include the virulence of the tubercle bacilli and characteristics of the alveolar macrophage such as their microbiocidal capacity. If large numbers of bacilli are present, the microbiocidal capacity of the nonsensitized macrophages may be exceeded, allowing the surviving organisms to multiply and establish a tuberculous infection (Hopewell, 1988; Nardell, 1993). If alveolar macrophages kill the tubercle bacilli at the time of the first exposure, then infection does not become established, and the tuberculin skin test remains negative as discussed in Chapter 8 (Pitchenik & Fertel, 1992).

Early after *M. tuberculosis* infection, an inflammatory response occurs within the lung. When this localized inflammation heals, a calcified parenchymal lesion called the primary or Ghon complex is left. Bacilli are still proliferating because cell mediated immunity has not developed (Dunlap & Briles, 1993) *M. tuberculosis* can replicate within the macrophages causing lysis, the escape of the tubercle bacilli and the infection of other alveolar macrophages (Edwards & Kirkpatrick, 1986; Moulding, 1983; Pitchenik et al., 1992).

At the time of the initial tuberculous infection, tubercle bacilli are transported within macrophages to regional lymph nodes in the hilum of the lung, ultimately allowing their entry into the bloodstream where the tubercle bacilli can then be seeded throughout the body, creating potential sites at which future extrapulmonary disease may develop. This lymphohematogenous dissemination of tubercle bacilli is usually asymptomatic; it occurs before the person acquires tuberculin hypersensitivity (Joklik, et al., 1992). Within the bloodstream, circulating tubercle bacilli are cleared by reticuloendothelial organs. However, bacterial multiplication continues in the lung apices where oxygen tension is high and the environment is favorable and in such areas as the kidneys, lymph nodes, and vascular skeletal areas such as the epiphyses (growing ends) of the long bones, all of which have favorable concentrations of oxygen (Joklik et al., 1992). Most of these lesions remain asymptomatic and heal with the development of cell-mediated immunity and delayed hypersensitivity that occur within a period of 3 to 8 weeks after infection, during which time the tuberculin skin test becomes reactive unless anergy (see Chapter 8) is present (Dunlap & Briles, 1993; Pitchenik et al., 1992).

At the time that the initial infection occurs, the immunologic defenses are stimulated but require 3 to 8 weeks to become effective (Joklik et al., 1992; Pitchenik et al., 1992). When the inhaled tubercle bacillus is phagocytized by the alveolar macrophage, mycobacterial antigens are released through lysis of the organisms. These antigens are processed by the macrophage and presented to the T-lymphocytes, which, in turn, proliferate and secrete mediators called lymphokines. The lymphokines include macrophage-activating factor, chemotactic factor, migration-inhibition factor, and mitogenic factor. The release of these mediators causes proliferation of lymphocytes and infiltration of the affected area with blood lymphocytes as well as monocytes that will become macrophages. These sensitized T and B lymphocytes and activated macrophages are much more effective at killing tubercle bacilli than the nonactivated macrophages that responded earlier to the initial infection (Edwards & Kirkpatrick, 1986; Hopewell, 1988; Moulding, 1983; Reynolds, 1987).

This acquired cell-mediated immunity constitutes the major determinant of host resistance to the further development of disease (Hopewell, 1988; Murray et al., 1990). The immunologic response kills bacteria and contains any remaining organisms by walling them off in a granulomatous tissue reaction (Daniel & Ellner, 1993; Joklik et al., 1992; Murray, 1989; Murray et al., 1990). The sequestered bacilli remain viable but become dormant, allowing the infection to remain latent as long as cell-mediated immunity remains intact. This tubercle formation or hypersensitivity granuloma is composed of macrophages and T cells that have been activated and responded to mycobacterial antigens, becoming enlarged, and often referred to as epithelioid cells. Often a peripheral collar of fibroblasts, macrophages, and lymphocytes surrounds it. Sometimes caseous necrosis occurs in the central part, and a "soft" tubercle results. These lesions may calcify, resulting in the primary or Ghon complex (Daniel & Ellner, 1993; Dunlap & Briles, 1993; Joklik et al., 1992; Kuritzkes & Simon, 1991). Should calcification of a hilar lymph node occur, this lesion and the Ghon complex collectively make up the Ranke complex (Edwards & Kirkpatrick, 1986; Hopewell, 1988; Moulding, 1983).

Of great clinical significance is whether the caseation necrosis remains a cheeselike consistency or whether it undergoes softening and liquefaction (Dannenberg, 1994). In the majority of people who are infected, after the tubercle is formed, the person is asymptomatic and infection is latent as the tubercle bacilli are dormant and contained by the immune system, and the tuberculin skin test will be positive. This is true in about 90% of exposed individuals. In some persons, however, cell-mediated immunity does not completely control primary tuberculosis, and liquefaction necrosis occurs with the primary infection evolving into clinical disease (Nardell, 1993). The mechanisms that cause liquefaction are unclear but when it occurs there is a massive increase in the number of tubercle bacilli. As liquefaction of a caseous mass occurs in the lung tissue, the liquefied material is expelled via the bronchi and a cavity forms. The number of bacilli in the resulting cavity will be very high probably because of the presence of softened caseum and a high concentration of oxygen, both of which are conducive to the growth of the organism (Joklik et al., 1992). Tuberculous pneumonitis may result, and patients with cavitary tuberculosis typically exhibit coughing and systemic symptoms such as fever, anorexia, and weight loss (Nardell, 1993). The consequences of this large population of bacilli existing in a cavity include the possibility of bronchogenic spread of bacilli to other portions of the lung and increased infectiousness of the infected person.

As previously stated, the adequacy of the immune response will determine whether tuberculous infection proceeds to disease. A relative minority of infected persons actually develop tuberculosis disease. Approximately 90% of infected individuals will remain free of clinical tuberculosis during their lifetime (Dunlap et al., 1993; Nardell, 1991). Of the remaining 10% of infected individuals, half of the total number of infected individuals (5%) will develop disease within the first few years after infection (early), whereas the remaining half will develop disease following a much longer interval (late), in some cases as long as several decades after the initial infection (Dunlap et al., 1993; Kuritzkes et al., 1991; Murray, 1989; Murray et al., 1990). Thus, in most cases the outcome for primary infection is control and resolution although viable bacilli can remain in the granulomas (and in other body sites) allowing reactivation if cell-mediated immunity is compromised. Typically, the only signs of resolved primary tuberculous infection are reactivity to the tuberculin skin test and sometimes chest radiographic evidence of the Ghon or Ranke complex (MacGregor, 1993).

The proper functioning of the elements involved in the immune response to *M. tuberculosis* as detailed above prevents progression to tuberculosis disease in the infected host and also boosts the immune response to any subsequent exposure to tubercle bacilli, thus preventing implantation and development of new infection. Any impairment of cell-mediated immunity creating an inadequate immune response, can, therefore, have the following possible consequences:

1. endogenous reactivation—reactivation of previously acquired tuberculous infection; or
2. exogenous infection or reinfection—acquisition of new infection with tubercle bacilli from an external source (Murray et al., 1990; Nardell, 1993).

Reactivation of a previously acquired tuberculous infection leading to clinical disease is most often seen after 50 years of age and is most common in males. This reactivation can result from a breakdown in cell-mediated immunity in the host from such causes as malnutrition, drug or alcohol use, diabetes, HIV-infection, other causes, and perhaps even severe stress (Sherris, 1990). These factors modify the immune response through their effects on the cells that initiate and modulate the immune response. In addition to the roles of other cell types in the acquisition of cell-mediated immunity, discussed earlier, subsets of the T-lymphocytes, the helper and suppressor cells, serve as regulators whose presence and activity determine the adequacy of the immune response (Moulding, 1983). The most common site for reactivation is in the apex of the lung where oxygen tension is high.

HIV INFECTION

Infection with the human immunodeficiency virus (HIV) is considered to be the greatest acquired risk factor for developing tuberculosis (Murray, 1989), and the increased incidence of TB in those with HIV infection is well documented (Heckbert, Elarth, & Nolan, 1992; Long, et al., 1991; Semenzato & Agostini, 1989; Shafer, Goldberg, Sierra, & Glatt, 1989). The major cellular immune defect in HIV infection is depletion of a specific subset of T-helper lymphocytes (T4 cells, CD4+ lymphocytes), but other elements of the immune system such as macrophages and monocytes may also be affected. These quantitative and qualitative immune impairments result in increased susceptibility to opportunistic infections and increased incidence of neoplasias (Cohen, 1993; Rosenberg & Fauci, 1991). Extrapulmonary TB has been an AIDS-defining condition in the United States, and the change in AIDS indicator conditions published in 1992 now includes pulmonary TB (Centers for Disease Control, 1987; Centers for Disease Control and Prevention, 1992).

Defenses against tuberculosis depend on an intact macrophage/mono-cyte-T-cell axis for development of an adequate immune response to the causative organism (Rankin, Collman, & Daniele, 1988; Reynolds, 1987). In the presence of HIV infection, there is unusual susceptibility to pulmonary infections caused by the *Mycobacterium* species, including *M. avium* complex, and tuberculosis (Agostini, Trentin, Zambello, & Semenzato, 1993). Development of tuberculosis disease in the HIV-infected individual occurs via the possible mechanisms previously dis-cussed—reactivation of latent TB infection and rapid progression of pri-mary exogenous acquired tuberculous infection to disease because of impaired cellular immunity, or exogenous reinfection rapidly leading to early disease (Pitchenik et al., 1992). Murray et al. (1990) state that because *M. tuberculosis* is relatively more virulent than other HIV-re-lated opportunistic pathogens that cause latent infection, it is often the first endogenous infection to reactivate as immunity is weakened due to HIV infection.

An increased incidence of multidrug-resistant tuberculosis in the HIV-infected and HIV-susceptible populations has also been noted (Busillo, et al., 1992; Chawla, Klapper, Kamholz, Pollack, & Heurich, 1992). Glassroth (1992) succinctly summarizes the implications of HIV infec-tion for the spread of tuberculosis. Where TB exists in a community, HIV-infected individuals within that community have the greatest risk of becoming infected and developing early disease. The disease process is accelerated, allowing less time for adequate treatment. In this way, the number of infectious persons within the community increases, thus increasing the likelihood of transmission of the organism to new hosts. It also increases the likelihood of the development of drug resistant strains of *M. tuberculosis*. If the infecting organisms are already drug resistant, it promotes the continued survival of the variant strain of or-ganism. This is further discussed in Chapters 3 and 5.

SUMMARY

Tuberculous infection and tuberculosis are the results of environmental exposure to the bacterial organism, *Mycobacterium tuberculosis*. Trans-mission in the U. S. is usually the result of inhalation of droplet nuclei containing tubercle bacilli. In primary infection, initially nonspecific responses and an inflammatory response occurs; after 3 to 8 weeks, delayed hypersensitivity and cell-mediated immunity develop and infec-tion is controlled. The pathogenesis involves contracting the infection, which may remain latent until (and if) activation occurs with the subse-quent development of tuberculosis. Risk factors for the development of tuberculosis include medications, diseases, age, malnutrition and genetic factors. The cause and pathogenesis of TB and the nature of the cellular defects of HIV infection make HIV-infected individuals particularly susceptible to the development of tuberculosis infection and disease, and it is now an AIDS-defining condition.

Tuberculosis is a chronic disease that can be controlled through proper case finding and treatment. The emergence of drug resistance in tuberculosis is of particular concern and requires that even more aggressive techniques be developed for disease control. Understanding the microbiology and pathogenesis of the disease process allows the clinician to understand the rationale for clinical interventions directed toward cure and prevention. The management of tuberculosis both in individual patients and as a major public health problem is discussed in the following chapters.

REFERENCES

Agostini, C., Trentin, L., Zambello, R., & Semenzato, G. (1993). HIV-1 and the lung: Infectivity, pathogenic mechanisms, and cellular immune responses taking place in the lower respiratory tract. *American Review of Respiratory Disease, 147,* 1038–1049.

American Thoracic Society. (1992). Control of tuberculosis in the United States. *American Review of Respiratory Disease, 146,* 1623–1633.

Busillo, C.P., Lessnau, K.D., Sanjana, V., Soumakis, S., Davidson, M., Mullen, M. P., & Talavera, W. (1992). Multidrug resistant Mycobacterium tuberculosis in patients with human immunodeficiency virus infection. *Chest, 102,* 797–801.

Centers for Disease Control (1987). Revision of the CDC surveillance case definition for the acquired immunodeficiency syndrome. *Morbidity and Mortality Weekly Report, 36(suppl 1S),* 1S–15S.

Centers for Disease Control. (1990). Screening for tuberculosis and tuberculous infection in high-risk populations. *Morbidity and Mortality Weekly Report, 39 (RR-8),* 1–7.

Centers for Disease Control and Prevention. (1992). 1993 revised classification system for HIV infection and expanded surveillance definition for AIDS among adolescents and adults. *Morbidity and Mortality Weekly Report,* 41(RR-17), 1–19.

Chawla, P.K., Klapper, P.J., Kamholz, S.L., Pollack, A.H., & Heurich, A.E. (1992). Drug resistant tuberculosis in an urban population including patients at risk for HIV infection. *American Review of Respiratory Disease., 146,* 280–284.

Clancy, L. (1990). Infectiousness of tuberculosis. *Bulletin of the International Union Against Tuberculosis and Lung Disease, 65,* 30.

Cohen, F. L. (1993). HIV infection and AIDS: An overview (pp. 3-30). In F. L. Cohen and J.D. Durham (Eds.). *Women, children and HIV/AIDS,* New York: Springer.

Constock, G. W., & Cauthen, G. M. (1993). Epidemiology of tuberculosis. *Lung Biology in health and Disease, 66,* 23–48.

Daniel, T. M. & Ellner, J. J. (1993). Immunology of tuberculosis. *Lung Biology in Health and Disease, 66,* 75–101.

Dannenberg, A. M. jr. (1994). Pathogenesis and immunology: Basic aspects. In D. Schlossberg (Ed). *Tuberculosis* (3rd ed), (pp. 17–39). New York: Springer-Verlag.

Dunlap, N. E. & Briles, D. E. (1993). Immunology of tuberculosis. *Medical Clinics of North America, 77,* 1235-1251.

Edwards, D. & Kirkpatrick, C.H. (1986). The immunology of mycobacterial disease. *American Review of REspiratory Disease, 134,* 1062–1071.

Glassroth, J. (1992). Tuberculosis in the United States: Looking for a silver lining among the clouds. *American Review of Respiratory Disease,146,* 278–279.

Grosset, J. H. (1993). Bacteriology of tuberculosis. *Lung Biology in Health and Disease, 66,* 49–74.

Heckbert, S.R., Elarth, A., & Nolan, C.M. (1992). The impact of human immunodeficiency virus infection on tuberculosis in young men in Seattle-King County, Washington. *Chest, 102,* 433–437.

Hopewell, P.C. (1988). Mycobacterial diseases. In J.F. Murray & J.A. Nadel (Eds.), *Textbook of respiratory medicine* (pp. 856–915). Philadelphia, PA.: W.B. Saunders.

Hopewell, P. C. (1993). Tuberculosis and infection with the human immunodeficiency virus. *Lung Biology in Health and Disease, 66,* 369–394.

Joklik, W. K., Willett, H. P., Amos, D. B., & Wilfert, C. M. (1992). *Zinsser microbiology,*(20th ed.). Norwalk, CT: Appleton & Lange.

Kramer, F., Sasse, S.A., Simms, J.C., & Leedom, J.M. (1993). Primary cutaneous tuberculosis after a needlestick injury from a patient with AIDS and undiagnosed tuberculosis. *Annals of Internal Medicine, 119,* 594–595.

Kuritzkes, D. R., & Simon, H. B. (1991). Pneumonia due to *M. tuberculosis* and to atypical mycobacteria. In J. Shelhamer, P. A. Pizzo, J. E. Parrillo & H. Masur (Eds). *Respiratory disease in the immunosuppressed host.* (pp.312–327). Philadelphia: J. B. Lippincott.

Long, R., Scalcini, M., Manfreda, J., Carrde,G., Philippe, E., Hershfield, E., Sekla, L., & Stackiw, W. (1991). Impact of human immunodeficiency virus type 1 on tuberculosis in rural Haiti. *American Review of Respiratory Disease, 143,* 69–73.

MacGregor, R. R. (1993). Tuberculosis: from history to current management. *Seminars in Roentgenology, XXVIII (2),* 101–108.

Mandell, G. L., Douglas, R. G. Jr., & Bennett, J. (Eds.). (1990). *Principles and Practice of Infectious Diseases.* (3rd ed.). New York: Churchill Livingstone.

Moulding, T. (1983). Pathogenesis, pathophysiology, and immunology. In D. Schlossberg (Ed.). *Tuberculosis: Vol.2 Praeger monographs in infectious disease* (pp. 21–35). New York: Praeger Publishers.

Moulding, T. (1994). Pathophysiology and immunology: Clinical aspects. In D. Schlossberg (Ed). *Tuberculosis* (3rd ed), (pp. 41–50). New York: Springer-Verlag.

Murray, J.F. (1989). The white plague: Down and out or up and coming. *American Review of Respiratory Disease, 140,* 1788–1795.

Murray, J.F. & Mills, J. (1990). Pulmonary infectious complications of human immunodeficiency virus infection. *American Review of Respiratory Disease, 141,* 1356–1372.

Nardell, E. A. (1990). Dodging droplet nuclei. *American Review of Respiratory Disease, 142,* 501–503.

Nardell, E. A. (1993). Pathogenesis of tuberculosis. *Lung Biology in Health and Disease, 66,* 103–122.

Pitchenik, A. E. & Fertel, D. (1992). Mycobacterial disease in patients with HIV infection. In G. P. Wormser (Ed.). AIDS and other manifestations of HIV infection (2nd ed., pp. 277–313). New York, Raven Press.

Rankin, J.A., Collman, R., & Daniele, R.P. (1988). Acquired immune deficiency syndrome and the lung. *Chest, 94,* 155–164.

Reynolds, H.Y. (1987). Host defense impairments that may lead to respiratory infections. *Clinics in Chest Medicine, 8* (3), 339–358.

Rosenberg, Z.F. & Fauci, A.S. (1991). Immunopathogenesis of HIV infection. *FASEB Journal., 5,* 2382–2390.

Riley, L. W. (1993). Drug-resistant tuberculosis. *Clinical Infectious Diseases,* 17 (Suppl 2), S441–S446. New York: Raven Press.

Shafer, R.W., Goldberg, R., Sierra, M. & Glatt, A.E. (1989). Frequency of Mycobacterium tuberculosis bacteremia in patients with tuberculosis in an area endemic for AIDS. *American Review of Respiratory Disease, 140,* 1611–1613.

Sherris, J. C. (Ed.).(1990). *Medical microbiology: an introduction to infectious diseases.* New York: Elsevier Science.

Semenzato, G. & Agostini, C. (1989). Human retroviruses and lung involvement. *American Review of Respiratory Disease, 139, 1317–1322.*

Witebsky, F. G., & Conville, P. S. (1993). The laboratory diagnosis of mycobacterial diseases. *Infectious Disease Clinics of North America, 7(2),* 359–376.

3

THE EPIDEMIOLOGY
OF TUBERCULOSIS

Felissa L. Cohen

Before the advent of AIDS and the recognition of HIV infection, it was a common misconception that infectious diseases had been all but eradicated. Worldwide, however, infectious diseases are still the leading cause of death, surpassing cardiovascular disease and cancer. Among the infectious diseases, tuberculosis (TB) is the leading cause of death in the world today (Bloom & Murray, 1992; Centers for Disease Control and Prevention, 1993c). In the United States in 1986 the number of reported TB cases per year showed an increase for the first time since recordkeeping began in 1953. DNA fingerprinting techniques have been used with traditional epidemiological methods to identify transmission patterns (Alland, Kalkut, Moss, et al., 1994; Small, Hopewell, Singh, et al., 1994). This chapter will discuss the epidemiology of TB in the United States and the world; multidrug-resistant TB; and the relationship of the dual epidemics of TB and human immunodeficiency virus (HIV) infection.

TABLE 3.1 TB Cases and Case Rates by Year in the United States*

Year	Number of Cases	Case Rate
1982	25,520	11.0
1983	23,846	10.2
1984	22,255	9.4
1985	22,201	9.3
1986	22,768	9.4
1987	22,517	9.3
1988	22,436	9.1
1989	23,495	9.4
1990	25,701	10.3
1991	26,283	10.4
1992	26,673	10.5
1993	25,313	9.8

*per 100,000 population

STATISTICS AND TRENDS IN THE UNITED STATES

In 1953 (the first year the Centers for Disease Control and Prevention [CDC] kept TB records) the number of reported TB cases in the United States was 84,304. Since that time, TB had been more or less steadily declining in the U.S. At times, this decline has slowed. For example, from 1975 to 1978, the average annual decrease in reported TB cases was 5.7%. From 1978 to 1981, the average decline was only 1.4%, a change that was attributed to the large influx of Southeast Asian refugees. The years from 1982 through 1984 showed a decline of 6.7%. In 1985, it was first observed that this decline had slowed to 2.0%, and 22,201 cases were reported (Centers for Disease Control, 1986a). In 1986, an increase was seen with 22,768 cases reported (Centers for Disease Control, 1988). In 1993, 25,313 cases of TB or 9.8 cases per 100,000 population were reported to CDC, a slight decrease from 1992 (Centers for Disease Control and Prevention, 1994b). The reasons for this overall decrease, while welcome, are not entirely clear. They may include the results of effective prevention and control measures, delayed reporting due to use of a new TB surveillance reporting form, or underreporting because of modification in the AIDS surveillance case definition, resulting in reporting of TB cases to AIDS surveillance but not TB surveillance for those who are coinfected with HIV and TB (Centers for Disease Control and Prevention, 1994b). The number of reported cases and case rates per 100,000 population of TB since 1982 are shown in Table 3.1.

Since it was observed that the TB decline trend had slowed, the cause

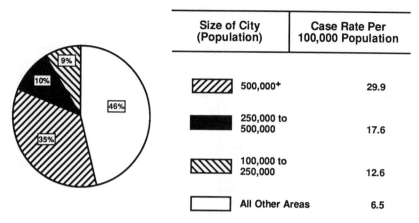

Size of City (Population)	Case Rate Per 100,000 Population
500,000+	29.9
250,000 to 500,000	17.6
100,000 to 250,000	12.6
All Other Areas	6.5

FIGURE 3.1 Tuberculosis cases in cities in the United States.

Source: Centers for Disease Control 1994c). *1992 tuberculosis statistics in the United States*. Atlanta, GA, U.S. Department of Health and Human Services, p. 83.

was thought to be what was then called human T-lymphotropic virus type III/lymphadenopathy-associated virus (HTLV-III/LAV) infection, now known as HIV infection (Centers for Disease Control, 1986a). However, although HIV infection is certainly a contributing factor to the rise in TB cases, other factors have probably also been important. These include the social conditions of poverty, crowding, poor nutrition, homelessness, drug use, and others; the deinstitutionalization of the mentally ill; increased immigration from countries with high prevalence rates of TB; previous relative apathy of the majority of both the public and professionals to TB; increasing costs of medication, and some shortages in their manufacture; and the decreased funding to support TB control programs in this country (Brudney & Dobkin, 1991; Joseph, 1993; Reichman, 1991).

Sites

In the United States, the majority (more than 80%) of TB cases are pulmonary. Extrapulmonary TB (EPTB) has remained relatively stable accounting for about 17% to 19% of the TB cases in the U.S. Among the extrapulmonary sites, lymphatic, pleural, bone and joint, and genitourinary are most common (Slutsker, Castro, Ward, & Dooley, 1993). EPTB appears more frequent among females than males in the United States, except for pleural TB (Rieder, Snider, & Cauthen, 1990). Extrapulmonary sites are relatively common in HIV infection and are discussed later in this chapter and in Chapter 5.

TABLE 3.2 U.S. Reported Tuberculosis Cases and Rates by Age, 1992

Age in Years	Cases No.	%	Case Rate (per 100,000)
0–4	1,074	4.0	5.5
5–14	633	2.4	1.7
15–24	1,975	7.4	5.5
25–35	5,073	19.0	11.9
35–44	5,380	20.2	13.5
46–54	3,635	13.6	13.3
55–64	2,861	10.7	13.7
65+	6,042	22.7	18.7
Total	26,673	100.0	—

Source: Centers for Disease Control and Prevention (1994c). *1992 Tuberculosis Statistics in the United States*. Atlanta, GA: U.S. Department of Health and Human Services.

Geographic Distribution

When unadjusted numbers of reported cases are examined by state, California, New York, Texas, Florida, and Illinois reported the most TB cases. When case rates per 100,000 population were examined in 1990, the highest rates were in New York, District of Columbia, Hawaii, California, Alabama, Georgia, Florida, New Jersey, Illinois, and Mississippi. The lowest case rates in 1992 were reported in Vermont, New Hampshire, Wyoming, North Dakota, and Iowa. Overall, the highest case rates were reported from cities with populations of 500,000 and more. However, nearly half of the number of cases was from cities with populations below 100,000. This distribution is shown in Figure 3.1. When cities with populations of 250,000 or more are examined according to case rate per 100,000 population in 1992, the highest rates are found in Atlanta, Georgia; Newark, New Jersey; New York, New York; San Francisco, California; and Miami, Florida. The greatest number of cases were reported from New York City, New York; Los Angeles, California; Chicago, Illinois; Houston, Texas; and San Francisco, California (Centers for Disease Control, 1994c). Many states and cities that have high rates of TB also have high rates of AIDS cases. For example, in New York City, 40% of those infected with TB are also HIV-infected (Goldsmith, 1993).

Age

Before the current resurgence in TB cases, TB had primarily been a disease of the elderly in the United States. The major reason for this

TABLE 3.3 U.S. Reported Tuberculosis Cases and Rates by Race/ Ethnicity

Race/Ethnicity	Cases: 1985 No.	%	Cases: 1992 No.	%	% Change
White, non-Hispanic	8,453	38.1	7,618	28.6	-9.9
African-American, non-Hispanic	7,592	34.2	9,623	36.1	+26.8
Hispanic	3,092	13.9	5,397	20.2	+74.5
Asian/Pacific Islander	2,530	11.4	3,698	13.9	+46.2
American Indian/Alaskan Native	397	1.8	305	1.1	-23.2
Unknown	137	0.6	32	0.1	
Total:	22,201		26,673		

Source: Center for Disease Control and Prevention (1993b). Tuberculosis morbidity—United States, 1992. *Morbidity and Morality Weekly Report, 42,* 696–697, 703–704.

pattern was that the majority of cases before 1985 were reactivation of old infections rather than newly acquired ones, and as the population aged and newly transmitted infections to younger persons decreased, it was the elderly in whom TB was most prevalent. It is estimated that 50 to 70 years ago 80% of all Americans had been infected with *Mycobacterium tuberculosis* by the age of 30 years. The persistence of that infection is said to account for 90% of the TB cases that occur in elderly persons (Dutt & Stead, 1992; Stead & Dutt, 1991).

In the United States, controlling for HIV infection, the TB case rate among those over 65 years of age is higher than for any other age group (Dutt & Stead, 1993; McDonald, 1993) (See Table 3.2). This is because, as discussed previously, tubercle bacilli remain viable after initial infection for years and are capable of causing active TB if conditions permit this to occur. Examples of such conditions include impairment of the immune system such as may occur with old age, with diseases such as diabetes mellitus, or with therapy such as with steroids. Although the elderly account for about 27% of the total U.S.-reported TB cases, this age group represents only 12.5% of the U. S. population (Centers for Disease Control, 1990). Further, primary TB may develop if a person is exposed to an active case of TB such as in a long-term care facility or nursing home. The TB case rate is 5 to 10 times higher among those elderly living in nursing homes than among those living at home. Healthy elderly persons living at home rarely develop TB (Stead & Dutt, 1991). TB in the elderly is considered further in Chapter 11, and in the next section on race/ethnicity.

Another vulnerable group is children. Between 1985 and 1992, the number of TB cases increased 36.1% in children under age 5, 34.1% in children aged 5–14 years, and 18.1% in those 15–24 years of age (Centers for Disease Control and Prevention, 1993b). In children, an increased prevalence of tuberculous infection was seen in international adoptees, which was in one study 100 times greater than in a comparable American population. American-born children at highest risk for TB are those who are black[1], Hispanic, or children of migrant farm workers, regardless of race or ethnicity (Goldsmith, 1990). Foreign-born cases represented 16% of children under 5 years of age with TB and 49% of adolescents 15 to 19 years of age with TB in 1990 (Jacobs & Starke, 1993). Tuberculous infection in the very young, particularly 6 months or younger, progresses to disease in high proportion (Mandell, Douglas, & Bennett, 1990). TB in children is considered further in Chapter 11.

Increases in TB cases in persons aged 25 to 44 years of age have been noted. Between 1985 and 1992, TB cases increased 54.5% in this group. A proportion of that increase could be attributed to the prevalence of HIV infection in that age group. Without considering sex, race, or ethnicity, the number and percent of TB cases in 1992 was highest for the 25-to-44 year age group, although the case rate was highest for those 65 years and older (Center for Disease Control and Prevention, 1993b). TB is now considered to be an increasing problem in women of reproductive age. In one review of medical records in the years 1985–1992 of two public hospitals in New York, 16 pregnant women with active TB were detected. The majority of those tested for HIV were HIV positive and 7 of the 16 currently used cocaine or heroin. Ten had pulmonary TB and the rest were extrapulmonary — tuberculous meningitis, mediastinal, renal, gastrointestinal, and pleural (Centers for Disease Control and Prevention, 1993a). TB in women and in pregnancy are considered in Chapter 11.

Race/Ethnicity

In 1990, nearly 70% of the adult and about 86% of TB cases in children below 15 years of age occurred among minorities, with non-Hispanic blacks at greatest risk, followed by Hispanics, Asians/Pacific Islanders and American Indians/Alaskan natives. Among both non-Hispanic blacks and Hispanics, increases in reported TB cases from 1985 to 1990 were

---

[1]Terms to refer to racial and ethnic groups are used in the way data are collected by the Centers for Disease Control and Prevention

TABLE 3.3 U.S. Reported Tuberculosis Cases and Rates by Race/Ethnicity

Race/Ethnicity	Cases: 1985 No.	%	Cases: 1992 No.	%	% Change
White, non-Hispanic	8,453	38.1	7,618	28.6	-9.9
African-American, non-Hispanic	7,592	34.2	9,623	36.1	+26.8
Hispanic	3,092	13.9	5,397	20.2	+74.5
Asian/Pacific Islander	2,530	11.4	3,698	13.9	+46.2
American Indian/Alaskan Native	397	1.8	305	1.1	-23.2
Unknown	137	0.6	32	0.1	
Total:	22,201		26,673		

Source: Center for Disease Control and Prevention (1993b). Tuberculosis morbidity—United States, 1992. *Morbidity and Morality Weekly Report, 42*, 696–697, 703–704.

greatest in the 5-to-14-year-old and 25-to-44-year-old age groups ("Prevention and Control . . . ", 1992b; Centers for Disease Control and Prevention, 1993a). In non-Hispanic whites in the United States, TB is still mainly a disease of the elderly whereas among minorities it is a disease of younger persons. For example, the median age of nonwhite TB cases was 39 years in 1989 as opposed to 61 years in non-Hispanic whites (McDonald, 1993). In the period from 1985 through 1992, both the change in the number of cases and the case rate increased in black, non-Hispanics, Hispanics, and Asian/Pacific Islanders; while decreasing in white, non-Hispanics, and American Indian/Alaskan Natives (Centers for Disease Control and Prevention, 1993a). The number and percent of TB cases by race/ethnicity are shown in Table 3.3. When age distribution and race are examined together without regard for HIV infection, in those 65 years of age and older, the number and percent distribution of TB cases is higher for whites than for nonwhites (31.2% vs. 16.8%); however the TB case rate per 100,000 population is higher for nonwhites (14.0 vs. 65.4, respectively) (Centers for Disease Control and Prevention, 1994c). (See Chapter 11). TB in Native Americans/Alaska native has declined from former highs, but they still bear a disproportionate burden of both tuberculous infection and tuberculosis. Moreover, there is a higher proportion of child and young adult cases in this group than in the United States at large. Although the most common form of TB is pulmonary among this group, there is a higher rate of certain types of extrapulmonary TB such as peritoneal TB. Additionally, this population has other risk factors such as a high prevalence of diabetes and a high

**TABLE 3.4 Estimated Number of Tuberculosis Cases[a] and Rates[b]—
Worldwide, 1990, 1995, 2000, and 2005**

Region	1990 Cases	Rate	1995 Cases	Rate	2000 Cases	Rate	2005 Cases	Rate
Southeast Asia	3,106	237	3,499	241	3,952	247	4,454	256
Western Pacific[c]	1,839	136	2,045	140	2,255	144	2,469	151
Africa	992	191	1,467	242	2,079	293	2,849	345
Eastern Mediterranean	641	165	745	168	870	168	987	170
Americas[d]	569	127	606	123	645	120	681	114
Eastern Europe[e]	194	47	202	47	210	48	218	49
Western Europe and others[f]	196	23	204	23	211	24	217	24
All regions	7,537	143	8,768	152	10,222	163	11,875	176
Percentage increase since 1990			*16.3%*		*35.6%*		*57.6%*	

[a]In Thousands
[b]Crude incidence rate per 100,000 population.
[c]Includes all countries of the World Health Organization's (WHO) Western Pacific region except Japan, Australia, and New Zealand.
[d] Includes all countries of WHO's American region except the United States and Canada.
[e]Includes all independent states of the former Union of Soviet Socialist Republics.
[f]Western Europe and the United States, Canada, Japan, Australia, and New Zealand.

Source: Centers for Disease Control and Prevention. (1993c) Estimates of future global tuberculosis morbidity and mortality from *Morbidity and Mortality Weekly Report, 42,* 962.

proportion of rapid acetylators of isoniazid (see Chapter 5). States reporting about three-quarters of TB cases in Native Americans are Arizona, Oklahoma, New Mexico, California, South Dakota, Washington, Montana, and Minnesota (Manfreda, Hershfield, Middaugh, Jones, & Breault, 1993).

WORLDWIDE STATISTICS

In April of 1993, the World Health Organization declared TB a global emergency ("WHO declares tuberculosis . . . ", 1993). The WHO TB program has estimated that about 1.7 billion people (or about one-third of the world population) had evidence of *M. tuberculosis* infection in 1990. Furthermore about 7.5 to 8 million new TB cases occur annually worldwide, and about 3 million deaths per year are attributed to TB

(McDonald, 1993). Nearly 5 million or two-thirds occurred in the Southeast Asian and Western Pacific regions. By the year 2005, it is estimated that the incidence of TB will increase to nearly 12 million cases per year, mainly because of an increase in AIDS. A sharp increase in both the number and case rate is projected for Africa by 2005. This information is shown in Table 3.4 (Centers for Disease Control and Prevention, 1993c). As is the case with many other disease statistics, accuracy in reporting varies widely among countries. In examining 15 western European countries in 1992, it has been recognized that, in several industrialized countries, declines in trends in reported TB has stabilized or reversed. In 1991, Portugal had the highest case rate while Denmark had the lowest ("Tuberculosis—Western Europe, 1974-1991," 1993).

The age distribution varies considerably between industrialized and developing countries. WHO estimates that 75% of tuberculous infected persons in developing countries are less than 50 years of age as compared with about 20% in developed countries. Developing countries also bear a disproportionate share of the mortality of TB; more than 98% of the approximate 3 million deaths per year is contributed by developing countries (Narain, Raviglione, & Kochi, 1992). It is estimated that between 8% and 20% of deaths due to TB in developing countries are in children (Starke, 1993).

GROUPS AT HIGH RISK FOR TUBERCULOSIS IN THE UNITED STATES

Some persons are at higher risk of TB than others either because they are more likely to be exposed to and infected by *Mycobacterium tuberculosis* or because once infected, they are more likely to progress to active tuberculosis (Centers for Disease Control, 1994b). Many of these are candidates for tuberculin skin testing programs (see Chapter 8). Groups known to have a higher prevalence of tuberculous infection include

- medically underserved populations (including some persons from minority groups);
- homeless persons;
- current or past prison inmates;
- alcoholics;
- injecting drug users;
- the elderly;
- foreign-born persons from countries with a high prevalence of TB;
- residents of long-term care facilities such as mental institutions and nursing homes; and

- contacts of TB cases.

Staff in hospitals, facilities where cough-inducing procedures such as pentamidine treatment for *Pneumocystis carinii* pneumonia (PCP), long-term care facilities, or any staff with prolonged contact with the above groups may also be at increased risk.

Groups having a higher risk of progression from tuberculous infection to active tuberculosis include

- persons who have recently acquired tuberculous infection (within the past 2 years);
- young children (5 years of age and less);
- persons with fibrotic lesions on chest radiograph; and
- those with certain medical conditions including HIV infection, silicosis, past gastrectomy or jejuno-ileal bypass surgery; chronic renal failure, diabetes mellitus, being 10% or more below ideal body weight, immunosuppression due to therapy with corticosteroids or other immunosuppressive drugs; and some malignancies (American Thoracic Society, 1992; Centers for Disease Control, 1990; Centers for Disease Control and Prevention, 1994b).

Circumstances and Medical Conditions That May Increase the Risk of Tuberculosis

Most of the medical conditions listed above act in some way to impair cell-mediated immunity, either directly or indirectly. For example, HIV infection results in depletion of the CD4+ cells and impairs immunity. Nutritional depletion or malnutrition can result in a lack of substances necessary for intact immune function leading to immune dysfunction. However, in some cases, the exact mechanism is not known. In the case of injecting drug users, multiple bouts of infection, the continuing injection of foreign substances into the body and poor nutrition may result in immune impairment (Cohen, 1991). In persons who abuse alcohol, it is thought that nutritional problems result in immune impairment, particularly cell-mediated responses (Hopewell, 1988). With both injecting drug users and alcoholics, social conditions such as homelessness may exacerbate the problem. In addition it has been noted that a lean body build has been associated with a higher risk of developing tuberculosis among those who were infected (Hoge, et al., 1994; Hopewell 1988). Men who were underweight in relation to their height had three times the rates of TB than others in one study (Hopewell, 1988). Also see Chapter 8.

Immigrants or Foreign-Born

A group at high-risk for TB in the United States are those persons born in countries with a high prevalence of TB. In the United States persons from six countries accounted for 63% of foreign-born TB cases. These were: China, Haiti, Mexico, the Phillipines, South Korea and Vietnam (Jacobs et al., 1993). In the majority of cases, it is within the first 5 years after arrival in the United States that TB is detected or identified. This means that following the health of these immigrants for 5 years could be useful. Reasons for difficulty in identification include those whose immigration is not legal; language and cultural barriers; poor access to care; difficulty in obtaining past medical records or documenting past tuberculin testing, vaccination, and/or treatment; poor adherence; difficulty in finding the person; poverty; mistrust of those in authority; fear and others (Jacobs et al., 1993; Orr & Hershfield, 1993). Immigration has played a major role in the increase of TB cases among women and children in the United States (Kent, 1993).

Socioeconomic Status

The association of TB with lower socioeconomic status has been well established and known for many decades. Contributory factors include homelessness, crowding, unclean living conditions, poor nutrition, decreased access to health care, and may be compounded by stress and substance abuse. It is still the trend today for poor immigrants from countries with high TB prevalence to come to large urban areas in the United States where TB risk among them may be high. This risk decreases with the longer duration of stay in this country (Comstock & Cauthen, 1993). Many who are disadvantaged socioeconomically are among the medically underserved. This group may disproportionately include racial and ethnic minorities. However, TB also occurs in those of middle and upper socioeconomic status.

TB In Jails, Prisons, and Correctional Institutions

Between 1985 and 1992, there were 11 reported TB outbreaks in prisons in eight states (Skolnick, 1993). A report in 1974 recognized that a stay in prison could contribute to the spread of TB in the surrounding community (Stead, 1974). More recent work has demonstrated that even 1 day in jail increases the risk for TB development. In many jails, inmates are initially held in crowded, poorly ventilated holding areas with others who have not been medically screened, thus creating high risk conditions for the acquisition of *M. tuberculosis*. In addition, intra-prison transmission of HIV infection through situational homosexuality or the use of injecting drugs can occur, leading to immunosuppression and susceptibility to the development of TB (Braun, 1993). When inmates are released to their communities, "they may bring an unanticipated burden from the correctional system to their wives, lovers, and children" (Bellin, Fletcher, & Safyer, 1993, p. 2231). Some correction facilities are now returning to chest x-ray screening because skin testing alone is ineffective in the correctional system particularly in those facilities where rapid shifting in populations occur (Skolnick, 1993). In addition to inmates, correctional system staff are also vulnerable to transmission. Another group exposed to the possibility of correctional facility-related transmission are attorneys, particularly public defenders who frequently visit their clients in jail.

TB Among Homeless Persons and in Shelters

Homelessness and congregate settings such as shelters and single-room occupancy hotels may also predispose to TB ("Prevention and Control of Tuberculosis Among Homeless . . . ", 1992a). Among those who live on the street and/or in shelters, medical disorders become magnified and exacerbated because of conditions of crowding, poor nutrition, exposure, stress resulting from fear of attack and concomitant physical conditions such as those resulting from long-term standing. Additionally, a proportion (many of whom would have been in psychiatric facilities before deinstitutionalization) are mentally ill, and about one-third are chronic substance abusers of alcohol, drugs, or both (Brickner, Scharer, & McAdam, 1993). In one report from a shelter in New York City, 42.8% of the homeless men evaluated were infected with TB, including 6% who had active TB. Among the independent risk factors identified were increasing age, minority group status, length of stay in shelter systems and intravenous drug use (McAdam, Brickner, Scharer, Crocco, & Duff, 1990). Nationally, the prevalence of latent TB infection among the homeless ranges from 18% to 51%, while active TB disease ranges from 1.6% to 6.8% (Prevention and Control of Tuberculosis Among Homeless . . . ", 1992a). It is estimated that the prevalence rates of active TB among the homeless are 150–300 times greater than in the general population (Brickner, et al., 1993). The problems of TB among the homeless and shelter residents is discussed further in Chapter 12.

TB In Rural and Farm Areas and Migrant Workers

Before 1990, despite lower case rates, small cities and rural areas accounted for more than half of the reported cases of TB in the United States (Robinson & Comstock, 1992). Since that time, they account for slightly less than half (Centers for Disease Control and Prevention, 1994c) (See Figure 3.1). Migrant farm workers are defined as "laborers whose principal employment is in agriculture on a seasonal basis and who establishes for the purposes of employment a temporary abode" (Centers for Disease Control, 1992a, p. 2). There are at least 4.2 million seasonal and migrant farm workers in the United States concentrated in three migrant stream patterns in the East, West, and Midwest (Centers for Disease Control, 1992a). Various studies of tuberculous infection prevalence have been carried out among migrant workers and have shown relatively high rates of infection. For example in one study in North Carolina, tuberculin positivity ranged from 33% (Hispanics) to 62% (blacks) to 76% (Haitians); while in another in Virginia, the overall rate in 1985 was 48% (Ciesielski, Seed, Esposito, & Hunter, 1991; Hibbs, Yeager, & Cochran, 1989). This group can be difficult to reach and to hold in treatment, and services should be provided by a team that includes an outreach worker from the same cultural and language background as the patients. The cost to employers and political issues impact upon TB service provisions to migrant farmworkers (Ciesielski, 1994). Tracking networks have been suggested as a means of facilitating follow-up care (Richard, 1994). The CDC have listed priority services with regard to TB for these workers and their families including children (Centers for Disease Control, 1992a).

GENETIC FACTORS

Although socioeconomic factors have been thought to be largely responsible for many racial/ethnic differences in TB, there also appears to be a role for genetic factors in resistance to TB infection. A study of more than 41,000 nursing home residents and of two prisons indicated that whites were more resistant than blacks with regard to initial infection with *Mycobacterium tuberculosis*. This resistance did not appear to extend to differences in progression to active clinical disease (Stead, Lofgren, Senner, & Reddick, 1990; Stead, 1992). In an in vitro study of macrophages among blacks and whites, it was found that the macrophages from black donors allowed more growth of the tubercle bacillus than did the macrophages from white donors. It was speculated that certain metabolites of Vitamin D might have some influence on this effect (Crowle & Elkins, 1990). In a study of schoolchildren exposed to a physical education teacher with active TB, white children were as susceptible as black children to TB infection. However, infected black children more frequently developed abnormal chest radiographs than did the infected white children (Hoge, et al., 1994). Afterschool exposures and previous TB status were unknown (Stead, Lofgren, & Senner, 1994). Other genetic factors and markers influencing TB resistance and susceptibility have been examined, including a greater concordance between identical than nonidentical twins, but no consistent associations have been noted.

OCCUPATIONAL RISK AND TB

Although TB is not usually considered as an occupational hazard, there are some situations in which occupation and TB are related. These include

1. Occupations including a large percentage of people at higher risk of TB—examples include unskilled workers such as laborers, food handlers, and custodial personnel;
2. Occupations increasing susceptibility to the development of TB—examples include mining, sandblasting, quarry work, and pottery;
3. Work settings that have the risk of increased exposure to TB—examples include hospitals, prisons, sites that administer aerosolized pentamidine, HIV clinics, residential mental health facilities, nursing homes, substance abuse treatment centers, homeless shelters, and mycobacteriology and other laboratories;
4. Work settings with relatively closed environments—examples include factories with reduced air circulation, submarines, airplanes, and so forth (Lanphear & Snider, 1991; Driver, Valway, Morgan et al., 1994).

HUMAN IMMUNODEFICIENCY VIRUS (HIV) INFECTION/AIDS AND TB

There are various lines of thinking that have supported the idea that the current HIV epidemic is one of the important reasons for the resurgence of TB in the United States (Styblo, 1991). These include the following: areas with the largest reported number of cases of AIDS have also had the greatest increases in reported cases of TB; those population groups with the highest AIDS prevalence have had the greatest increases in TB incidence; the incidence of TB among persons with AIDS is much higher than in the general population; and the immunologic impairments caused by HIV can result in the inability to contain previous infection with *Mycobacterium tuberculosis* or may not control a new infection (Barnes, Bloch, Davidson, & Snider, 1991; Daley, et al., 1992).

The connection between TB and HIV has been summarized by James Curran at CDC as "TB and HIV like to hang out together and they're a bad influence on each other." (HIV-Related Tuberculosis, 1992, p. 7). Extrapulmonary and disseminated TB (EPTB) have been AIDS-defining conditions since the 1987 revision of the CDC definition (Centers for Disease Control, 1987). But it was not until the most recent revision of the AIDS surveillance definition and classification system that pulmonary tuberculosis coupled with CD4+ counts <200 mm³, was added as an AIDS-defining condition (Centers for Disease Control and Prevention, 1992c). Worldwide about 3.1 to 3.5 million people are infected with both HIV and TB (Barnes & Barrows, 1993; "WHO declares tuberculosis . . . ", 1993).

There are two ways in which HIV-infected persons commonly acquire TB — through reactivation of a previous and latent infection or through new exposure to *Mycobacterium tuberculosis* with clinical disease developing quickly because of inability to contain infection (Daley et al., 1992). Recent studies indicate that the latter manner of acquisition and progression may be more common than formerly thought (Hamburg & Frieden, 1994). In many cases the appearance of TB in those already infected with HIV precedes the recognition of their HIV infection, although it can, of course, follow it (Centers for Disease Control, 1989). For example, in Florida, 57% of a series of 109 patients with AIDS developed TB more than 1 month before the diagnosis of AIDS was made (Centers for Disease Control, 1986b). A CDC survey of TB clinics across the United States revealed HIV-seropositivity rates of 0 to 46%, depending on geographic location. Thus, health care providers working with patients who have TB should maintain a high index of suspicion for HIV infection, particularly for those with unusual clinical features, and those working with HIV-infected patients should consider the possibility of TB. Health care workers caring for persons with HIV may be at risk for acquiring TB if appropriate infection control procedures are not followed (Di Perri, et al., 1992). TB in HIV-infected patients may have a course that rapidly progresses to active, infectious TB adding to the risk of transmission (Edlin, et al., 1992). Aerosolized pentamidine treatment for *Pneumocystis carinii* pneumonia (PCP), for example, can result in the release of many infectious particles into the air in patients with active TB, particularly if not identified. Special precautions for such administration are necessary (see Chapter 9). Furthermore, as discussed in Chapter 8, anergy due to the impairment of cell-mediated immunity makes routine tuberculin skin testing less than reliable in those who are HIV-infected, so anergy testing should be done, or other diagnostic methods used.

TB in persons with HIV infection may have a different clinical presentation than those whose cellular immunity is normal. This is true of both pulmonary and extrapulmonary TB (Centers for Disease Control, 1989). Extrapulmonary sites for TB are estimated to occur in more than 70% of persons with TB and pre-existing AIDS and 24% to 45% of those with TB and less-advanced HIV infection (Slutsker, et al., 1993). It may also be combined with pulmonary TB. When TB occurs before another opportunistic infection in people with HIV infection, between 75 and 100% will have pulmonary TB (Yamaguchi & Reichman, 1991). Because TB is the most common infection in persons with HIV disease that is preventable, transmissible, and curable, health professionals have an opportunity for meaningful action.

MULTIDRUG-RESISTANT TUBERCULOSIS

One of the most-feared occurrences in the recent resurgence of TB has been the outbreaks and spread of multidrug-resistant (MDR) TB. MDR-TB has been called the third epidemic (Neville, et al., 1994). Although MDR-TB has been variously defined, CDC has considered it to include those organisms that were resistant to at least isoniazid and rifampin ("Nosocomial transmission of multidrug-resistant . . . ," 1990). Drug resistance in disease and in TB were known earlier. Between the years of 1975 and 1982, CDC monitored the prevalence of primary drug-resistant TB defined below. The rates decreased from 13% to 7% in that time period and increased to 9% in 1986. Most of these drug-resistant strains were resistant to single drugs, usually isoniazid or streptomycin (Wolinsky, 1993). From 1982 to 1985, only 0.5% of new TB cases were resistant to both isoniazid and rifampin (two of the most effective drugs for TB); but by 1991, this had risen to 3.1% for new cases and 6.9% for recurrent cases, and overall in 1991, 14.4% of the TB cases tested had organisms resistant to at least one anti-TB drug. In New York City, 33% of TB cases tested had organisms resistant to at least one drug, and in 19% of cases they were resistant to both isoniazid and rifampin (Centers for Disease Control, 1992b). Geography appears to be the major risk factor for MDR-TB, and the greatest problem exists in New York City (Bloch, et al., 1994).

Several types of drug resistance may occur. These include patients who have a strain of organism that is naturally resistant before any drugs are given (primary), patients who acquire a drug-resistant strain from another patient, and drug resistance that results from treatment-related causes (Riley, 1993; Small, et al., 1993). In the latter case, treatment with a single medication or an ineffective drug regimen can result in the occurrence of drug-resistant mutants that can multiply and become significant in the patient's infection, becoming dominant (Goble, 1986). Because the mutation rate is usually in the order of 1 in 10^6 to 1 in 10^8 for isoniazid and for rifampin, respectively, the probability for a patient to have sufficient resistant organisms to be problematic is low; however, if those susceptible to a given drug are eliminated, then resistant mutants can grow and even become predominant (Goble, 1986). By giving two (or more) drugs simultaneously, the theory is that some organisms that may be resistant to the first drug will be susceptible to the second drug and vice-versa. The addition of a third or more drug provides an even greater safety net (Iseman & Madsen, 1989; Riley, 1993). Incorrect drug administration or nonadherence to therapy can also result in the development of drug-resistant strains. Sometimes patients are partially adherent to therapy, either missing doses or eliminating one in a series of medications they are taking for tuberculosis. The major risk factors for the development of MDR-TB are discussed in Chapter 5.

Nosocomial Transmission

Nosocomial transmission of TB from patient-to-patient, patient-to-health care workers, and patient-to-visitors has been documented for decades and have recently been seen generally and in units with HIV-infected patients (Dooley, et al., 1992). The chief reasons include lapses in infection control procedures, inadequate isolation techniques, and in delays in diagnosis, drug-susceptibility testing, and adequate therapy (Kent, 1993). Such transmission has become even more dangerous in the era of MDR-TB. Outbreaks of MDR-TB in institutional settings such as hospitals and correctional facilities have been investigated beginning in 1990, but began to occur in early 1988 ("Nosocomial transmission of multi-drug resistant tuberculosis . . . ", 1990). These sites were in Florida and New York, and more than 200 persons have been affected; most were also HIV-infected (Centers for Disease Control, 1991; Centers for Disease Control, 1992b). San Francisco has also reported outbreaks. Mortality has been high, ranging from 72% to 89%, with some patients having organisms resistant to seven anti-TB drugs. In addition, the median time interval between diagnosis with TB and death was as short as 4 to 16 weeks. Some health care and correctional workers in these facilities have acquired MDR-TB infection resulting in active disease and

CHESTER COLLEGE LIBRARY

death. In addition to factors discussed above regarding the emergence of MDR-TB, CDC states that some areas lack proper facilities and practices for controlling TB transmission, and drug susceptibility tests have taken time to perform with treatment and management not always being effective (Centers for Disease Control, 1992b). Adhering to appropriate infection control procedures is vital for reducing the transmission of TB within institutions. Conducting serial testing with the two-step method and annually thereafter and realizing that conversions of tuberculin tests in staff can serve as a marker for TB transmission within the health care facility are ways to assess the adequacy of infection control within the facility and recognize conversions quickly (Adler, 1993; Dooley, et al., 1992). For staff in high risk areas such as active TB units or units with HIV-positive patients, some recommend tuberculin skin testing every 3 to 6 months (Center for Disease Control and Prevention, 1994b; Kent, 1993). Tuberculin skin testing for those in hospitals should include students, physicians with admitting privileges, house staff, and volunteers. No group should be excluded. It is vital to prevent nosocomial transmission of TB. There is no contraindication to repeat tuberculin skin testing if the previous test was negative (Adler, 1993).

SUMMARY

Tuberculosis continues to increase in the United States and throughout the world. More cases mean more opportunities for a given individual to be in contact with someone who has infectious TB. The greatest increase in cases in this country is seen in urban dwellers, minorities, people from countries with high TB prevalence, the socioeconomically disadvantaged, substance abusers, the 25 to 44 age group, and those who are HIV-infected. Cases are also increasing in children and adolescents under 15 years of age in the United States and in developing countries. Multidrug-resistant TB poses new challenges because of its high rate of transmission to health care and other workers and its high fatality rate.

REFERENCES

Adler, J.J. (1993). Hospital-aquired tuberculosis: Addressing the challenge. *Hospital Practice, 28* (9), 109–120.
Allard, D., Kalkut, G. E., Moss, A. R., McAdam, R. A., Hahn, J. A., Bos-

worth, W., Drucker, E., & Bloom, B. R. (1994). Transmission of tuberculosis in New York City. *New England Journal of Medicine, 330,* 1710–1716.

American Thoracic Society. (1992). Control of tuberculosis in the United States. *American Review of Respiratory Disease, 146,* 1623–1633.

Barnes, P. F., & Barrows, S. A. (1993). Tuberculosis in the 1990s. *Archives of Internal Medicine, 119,* 400–410.

Barnes, P. F., Bloch, A. B., Davidson, P. T., & Snider, S. E., Jr. (1991). Tuberculosis in patients with human immunodeficiency virus infection. *New England Journal of Medicine, 324,* 1644–1650.

Bellin, E. Y., Fletcher, D. D., & Safyer, S. M. (1993). Association of tuberculosis infection with increased time in or admission to the New York City jail system. *Journal of the American Medical Association, 269,* 2228–2231.

Bloch, A. B., Cauthen, G. M., Onorato, I. M., Dansbury, K. G., Kelly, G. D., Driver, C. R., & Snider, D. E. Jr. (1994). Nationwide survey of drug-resistant tuberculosis in the United States. *Journal of the American Medical Association, 271,* 665–671.

Bloom, B. R., & Murray, C. J. L. (1992). Tuberculosis: Commentary on a reemergent killer. *Science, 257,* 1055–1064.

Braun, M. M. (1993). Tuberculosis in correctional facilities. *Lung Biology in Health and Disease, 66,* 551–570.

Bricker, P. W., Scharer, L. L., & McAdam, J. M. (1993). Tuberculosis in homeless populations. *Lung Biology in Health and Disease, 66,* 433–454.

Brudney, K., & Dobkin, J. (1991). Resurgent tuberculosis in New York City. *American Review of Respiratory Disease, 144,* 745–749.

Centers for Disease Control. (1986a). Tuberculosis—United States, 1985—and the possible impact of human T-lymphotropic virus type III/lymphadenopathy-associated virus infection. *Morbidity and Mortality Weekly Report, 35,* 74–76.

Centers for Disease Control (1986b). Tuberculosis and acquired immunodeficiency syndrome—Florida. *Morbidity and Mortality Weekly Report, 35,* 587–590.

Centers for Disease Control. (1987). Revision of the CDC surveillance case definition for the acquired immunodeficency syndrome. *Morbidity and Mortality Weekly Report, 36(suppl 1S),* 1S–15S.

Centers for Disease Control. (1988). Tuberculosis, final data—United States, 1986. *Morbidity and Mortality Weekly Report, 36,* 817–820.

Centers for Disease Control. (1989). Tuberculosis and human immunodeficiency virus infection: recommendations of the Advisory Committee for the Elimination of Tuberculosis (ACET). *Morbidity and Mortality Weekly Report, 38,* 236–250.

Center for Disease Control. (1990). Prevention and control of tuberculosis in facilities providing long-term care to the elderly. *Morbidity and Mortality Weekly Report, 39 (RR-10),* 7–13.

Centers for Disease Control (1991). Nosocomial transmission of multidrug-resistant tuberculosis among HIV-infected persons—Florida and New York, 1988–1991. *Morbidity and Mortality Weekly Report, 40,* 585–591.

Centers for Disease Control. (1992a). Prevention and control of tuberculosis in migrant farm workers. *Morbidity and Mortality Weekly Report, 41(RR–10)*, 1–15.

Centers for Disease Control. (1992b) National action plan to combat multidrug-resistant tuberculosis. *Morbidity and Mortality Weekly Report, 41(No.RR–11)*, 1–48.

Centers for Disease Control and Prevention. (1992c). 1993 revised classification system for HIV infection and expanded surveillance definition for AIDS among adolescents and adults. *Morbidity and Mortality Weekly Report, 41(RR–17)*, 1–19.

Centers for Disease Control and Prevention. (1993a). Tuberculosis among pregnant women—New York City, 1985–1992. *Morbidity and Mortality Weekly Report, 42*, 605, 611–612.

Centers for Disease Control and Prevention (1993b). Tuberculosis morbidity—United States, 1992. *Morbidity and Mortality Weekly Report, 42*, 696–704.

Centers for Disease Control and Prevention (1993c). Estimates of future global tuberculosis morbidity and mortality. *Morbidity and Mortality Weekly Report, 42*, 961–964.

Centers for Disease Control and Prevention (1994a). Expanded tuberculosis surveillance and tuberculosis morbidity—United States, 1993. *Morbidity and Mortality Weekly Report, 43*, 361–366.

Centers for Disease Control. (1994b). Guidelines for preventing the transmission of *Mycobacterium tuberculosis* in health-care facilities, 1994. *Morbidity and Mortality Weekly Report, 43* (RR-13), 1–133.

Centers for Disease Control and Prevention. (1994c) *1992 tuberculosis statistics in the United States.* Atlanta, GA, U.S. Department of Health and Human Services.

Ciesielski, S.D., Seed, J.R., Esposito, P.H. & Hunter, N. (1991). The epidemiology of TB among North Carolina migrant farm workers. *Journal of the American Medical Association, 265*, 1715–1719.

Cohen, F. L. (1991). The etiology and epidemiology of HIV infection and AIDS. In: J.D. Durham & F.L. Cohen (Eds.), *The person with AIDS: Nursing perspectives.* 2nd ed.) (pp.1–59). New York: Springer.

Comstock, G. W., & Cauthen, G. M. (1993). Epidemiology of tuberculosis. *Lung Biology in Health and Disease, 66*,23–48.

Crowle, A. J., & Elkins, N. (1990). Relative permissiveness of macrophages from black and white people for virulent tubercle bacilli. *Infection and Immunology, 58*, 632–638.

Daley, C. L., Small, P. M., Schechter, G. F., Schoolnik, G. K., McAdam, R. A., Jacobs, W. R. Jr., & Hopewell, P. C. (1992). An outbreak of tuberculosis with accelerated progression among persons infected with the human immunodeficiency virus. *New England Journal of Medicine, 326*, 231–235.

Di Perri, G., Cadeo, G. P., Castelli, F., Cazzadori, A., Bassetti, S., Rubini, F., Micciolo R., Concia, E. & Bassetti, D. (1992). Transmission of HIV-associated tuberculosis to health care workers. *Lancet, 340*, 682.

Dooley, S. W., Villarino, M.E., Lawrence, M., Salinas, L., Amil, S., Rullan,

J.V., Jarvis, W.R., Bloch, A.B. & Cauthen, G. M. (1992). Nosocomial transmission of tuberculosis in a hospital unit for HIV-infected patients. *Journal of the American Medical Association, 267,* 2632-2635.

Driver, C. R., Valway, S. E., Morgan, W. M., Onorato, I. M., & Castro, K. G. (1994). Transmission of *Mycobacterium tuberculosis* associated with air travel. *Journal of the American Medical Association, 272,* 1031-1035.

Dutt, A. K., & Stead, W. W. (1992). Tuberculosis. *Clinics in Geriatric Medicine, 8,* 761-775.

Dutt, A. K., & Stead, W. W. (1993). Tuberculosis in the elderly. *Medical Clinics of North America, 77*(6), 1353-1368.

Edlin, B.R., Tokars, J.I., Grieco, M.H., Crawford, J.T., Williams, J., Sordillo, E.M., Ong, K.R., Kilburn, J.O., Dooley, S.W., Castro, K.G., Jarvis, W.R., & Holmberg, S.D. (1992). An outbreak of multidrug-resistant tuberculosis among hospitalized patients with the acquired immunodeficiency syndrome. *New England Journal of Medicine, 326,* 1514-1521.

Goble, M. (1986). Drug-resistant tuberculosis. *Seminars in Respiratory Medicine, 1,* 220-229.

Goldsmith, M.F. (1990). Forgotten (almost) but not gone, tuberculosis looms large on domestic scene. *Journal of the American Medical Association, 264,* 165-166.

Goldsmith, M. F. (1993). New reports make recommendations, ask for resources to stem TB epidemic. *Journal of the American Medical Association, 269,* 187-191.

Hamburg, M. A., & Frieden, T. R. (1994). Tuberculosis transmission in the 1990s. *New England Journal of Medicine, 330,* 1750-1751.

Hibbs, J., Xeager, S.,& Cochran, J. (1989). Tuberculosis among migrant farm workers. *Journal of the American Medical Association, 262,* 1775.

HIV-related tuberculosis. Narrative text. (1992). Atlanta: Centers for Disease Control.

Hoge, C. W., Fisher, L., Donnell, H. D. Jr., Dodson, D. R., Tomlinson, G. V. Jr., Breiman, R. R., Bloch, A. B., & Good, R. C. (1994). Risk factors for transmission of *Mycobacterium tuberculosis* in a primary school outbreak: lack of racial difference in susceptibility to infection. *American Journal of Epidemiology, 139,* 520-530.

Hopewell, P. C. (1988). Mycobacterial diseases. In J.F. Murray, & J. A. Nadel (Eds.), *Textbook of respiratory medicine* (pp. 856-915), Philadelphia: W. B. Saunders.

Iseman, M. D., & Madsen, L. A. (1989). Drug-resistant tuberculosis. *Clinics in Chest Medicine, 10,* 341-353.

Jacobs, R. F. & Starke, J. R. (1993). Tuberculosis in children. *Medical Clinics of North America, 77*(6), 1335-1351.

Joseph, S. (1993). Editorial: Tuberculosis, again. *American Journal of Public Health, 83,* 647-648.

Kent, J. H. (1993). The epidemiology of multidrug-resistant tuberculosis in the United States. *Medical Clinics of North America, 77,* 1391-1409.

Lanphear, B. P., & Snider, D. E. Jr. (1991). Myths of tuberculosis. *Journal of Occupational Medicine, 33,* 501-504.

Mandell, G. L., Douglas, R. G. Jr., & Bennett, J. (Eds.). (1990). *Principles and Practice of Infectious Diseases*. (3rd ed.). New York: Churchill Livingstone.

Manfreda, J., Hershfield, E.S., Middaugh, J. P., Jones, M.E., & Breault, J.L. (1993). Tuberculosis in native North Americans. *Lung Biology in Health and Disease*, *66*, 455–482.

McAdam, J. M., Brickner, P.W., Scharer, L. L., Crocco, J. A., & Duff, A. E. (1990). The spectrum of tuberculosis in a New York City men's shelter clinic (1982–1988). *Chest*, *97*, 798–805.

McDonald, R. J. (1993). Tuberculosis in the elderly. *Lung Biology in Health and Disease*, *66*, 413–432.

Narain, J. P., Raviglione, M. C., & Kochi, A. (1992). HIV-associated tuberculosis in developing countries: Epidemiology and strategies for prevention. Geneva: World Health Organization, WHO/TB/92.164.

Neville, K., Bromber, A., Bromberg, R., Bonk, S., Hanna, B. A., & Rom, W. N. (1994). The third epidemic—multidrug-resistant tuberculosis. *Chest*, *105*, 45–48.

Nosocomial transmission of multidrug-resistant tuberculosis to health-care workers and HIV-infected patients in an urban hospital —Florida. (1990). *Morbidity and Mortality Weekly Report*, *39*, 718–722.

Orr, P. H., & Hershfield, E. S. (1993). The epidemiology of tuberculosis in the foreigh-born in Canada and the United States. *Lung Biology in Health and Disease*, *66*, 531–550.

Prevention and Control of Tuberculosis Among Homeless Persons. Recommendations of the Advisory Council for the Elimination of Tuberculosis. (1992a). *Morbidity and Mortality Weekly Report*, *41*(No. RR–5), 13–23.

Prevention and Control of Tuberculosis in U.S. Communities with At-Risk Minority Populations. Recommendations of the Advisory Council for the Elimination of Tuberculosis.(1992b). *Morbidity and Mortality Weekly Report*, *41*(No. RR–5), 1–11.

Reichman, L. B. (1991). The U-shaped curve of concern. *American Review of Respiratory Disease*, *144*, 741–742.

Reichman, L. B. (1993). Fear, embarrassment, and relief: The tuberculosis epidemic and public health. *American Journal of Public Health*, *83*, 639–641.

Richard, J. R. (1994). TB in migrant farmworkers. *Journal of the American Medical Association*, *271*, 905.

Rieder, H.L., Snider, D.E. Jr., & Cauthen, G.M. (1990). Extrapulmonary tuberculosis in the United States. *American Review of Respiratory Disease*, *141*, 347–351.

Riley, L. W. (1993). Drug-resistant tuberculosis. *Clinical Infectious Diseases*, *17 (Suppl 2,)*, S442–S446.

Robinson, D. B., & Comstock, G. W. (1992). Tuberculosis in a small semi-rural county. *Public Health Reports*, *107*, 179–182.

Skolnick, A. A. (1993). Correction facility TB rates soar; some jails bring back chest roentgenograms. *Journal of the American Medical Association*, *268*, 3175–3176.

Slutsker, L., Castro, K. G., Ward, J. W., & Dooley, S. W. Jr. (1993). Epidemiology of extrapulmonary tuberculosis among persons with AIDS in the United States. *Clinical Infectious Diseases, 16*, 513–518.

Small, P.M., Shafer, R.W., Hopewell, P.C., Singh, S.P., Murphy, M.J., Desmond, E., Sierra, M.F., & Schoolnik, G.K. (1993). Exogenous reinfection with multidrug-resistant *Mycobacterium tuberculosis* in patients with advanced HIV infection. *New England Journal of Medicine, 328*, 1137–1144.

Small, P.M., Hopewell, P. C., Singh, S. P., Paz, A., Parsonnet, J., Ruston, D. C., Schecter, G. F., Daley, C. L., & Schoolnik, G. K. (1994). The epidemiology of tuberculosis in San Francisco. *New England Journal of Medicine, 330*, 1703–1709.

Starke, J. R. (1993). Tuberculosis in children. *Lung Biology in Health and Disease, 66*, 329–367.

Stead, W. W. (1974). Undetected tuberculosis in prison: Source of infection for community at large. *Journal of the American Medical Association, 240*, 2544–2547.

Stead, W. W. (1992). Genetics and resistance to tuberculosis. Could resistance be enhanced by genetic engineering? *Annals of Internal Medicine, 116*, 937–941.

Stead, W. W. & Dutt, A. K. (1991). Tuberculosis in elderly persons. *Annual Review of Medicine, 42*, 267–276.

Stead, W. W., Lofgren, J. P., Senner, J. W., & Reddick, W. T. (1990). Racial differences in susceptibility to infection with *M. tuberculosis*. *New England Journal of Medicine, 322*, 422–427.

Stead, W. W., Lofgren, J. P., & Senner, J. W. (1994). Invited commentary: Relative susceptibility of black Americans to tuberculosis. *American Journal of Epidemiology, 139*, 531–532.

Styblo, K. (1991). The impact of HIV infection on the global epidemiology of tuberculosis. *Bulletin of the International Union of Tuberculosis and Lung Diseases, 66*, 27–32.

Tuberculosis—Western Europe, 1974–1991.(1993). *Morbidity and Mortality Weekly Report, 42*, 628–631.

WHO declares tuberculosis a global emergency. Press release WHO/31, Geneva, April 23, 1993.

Wolinsky, E. (1993). Statement of the tuberculosis committee of the Infectious Diseases Society of America. *Clinical Infectious Diseases, 16*, 627–628.

Yamaguchi, E., & Reichman, L. B. (1991). Pulmonary tuberculosis in the HIV-positive patients. *Infectious Disease Clinics of North America, 5*, 623–633.

PART II
Clinical Management
of Tuberculosis

4

SYMPTOMS AND DIAGNOSIS OF TUBERCULOSIS

Felissa L. Cohen, Carol D. Harriman, and Lorie Madsen*

Detection by tuberculin testing, recognition of the clinical presentation, and timely diagnosis are the essential first steps in successful treatment of infection or disease due to *Mycobacterium tuberculosis*. These steps are often made difficult by social conditions, such as homelessness, and concurrent disease, such as HIV/AIDS. In those with HIV disease or other immunodeficiency states, TB may present atypically, and diagnosis may be delayed leading to prolonged infectiousness and life-threatening disease. This chapter will discuss the clinical presentation of TB and the procedures required to make a diagnosis.

**Authors are listed alphabethically as equal contributors.

SYMPTOMS AND ASSESSMENT

Recognizing and diagnosing TB combines the assessment of the clinical symptoms, patient history, the physical examination, prior and current tuberculin test status, patient risk status, chest x-ray, and sputum examination. Pulmonary TB is the major type of TB seen among adults in the U.S. although as noted previously, any organ system may be involved. Symptoms may vary with the specific organ affected.

Presentation of Pulmonary Tuberculosis

In those who are not HIV-infected, the usual clinical presentation of pulmonary tuberculosis is insidious, with gradual development of vague symptoms. Other types of presentations include an onset initially characterized by cough and followed by other symptoms; an onset characterized by hemoptysis; one in which pleuritic pain predominates; and an acute onset characterized as flulike (Wolinsky, 1988). Common symptoms include

- cough, usually productive, occasionally with blood-streaked sputum;
- fatigue or malaise;
- anorexia;
- weight loss;
- low grade fever, often occurring in the afternoon—may be intermittent
- sweating and/or chills at night; and
- dull, aching chest pain or tightness (MacGregor, 1993; Schluger & Rom, 1994; Wolinsky, 1988).

All of the above symptoms may not be present, and the severity of a particular symptom may be variable. A general rule of thumb is to suspect TB in any patient with any ill-defined respiratory disease process. Fever, if present, is usually more common in the late afternoon and evening. Night sweats can be drenching, requiring a change in bedding or night clothes. Weight loss is common, despite adequate intake, owing to the increased catabolic state associated with disease. Dyspnea is not commonly seen. Rales may be heard near the apex of the lung. Laboratory abnormalities may be relatively nonspecific if present and can include anemia, elevated sedimentation rate, and a normal white blood cell count with monocytosis (Hopewell, 1988; MacGregor, 1993). Symptoms may be subtle as is common in the elderly (Couser & Glassroth,

TABLE 4.1 Major Sites and Symptoms of Extrapulmonary Tuberculosis

Site or Type	Major Signs and Symptoms
Lymphatic	Enlarged, usually non-painful lymph nodes
Renal	Hematuria, dysuria, pyuria, pain
Tuberculous meningitis	Headache, change in mentation and behavior, convulsions
Pericardial	Effusion, fever, pericardial pain
Vertebral	Pain, vertebral deformity, abscess, paralysis
Peripheral skeleton	Pain, soft tissue swelling, bony tissue destruction
Male genitalia	Scrotal mass, beaded vas deferens, draining scrotal sinus, pain, oligospermia
Female reproductive organs	Abdominal pain, menstrual disorders, infertility
Abdominal/intestinal	Pain, diarrhea, constipation, loss of weight, anorexia, abdominal mass
Larynx	Hoarseness, sore throat, cough*
Skin	Granulomatous skin lesions, deep tissue penetration
Miliary	Low-grade fever, fatigue, weakness, anorexia, weight loss, hepatomegaly, lymphadenopathy, choroidal tubercles, cough

*Note: These patients are highly infectious

1993) or may be attributed to other illness, such as in those with HIV-infection. Thus, the clinician must entertain the possibility of tuberculosis when confronted by a patient with even a few of the classic symptom even if nonspecific.

Presentation of Extrapulmonary Tuberculosis

Virtually any organ can be infected with TB. TB in organ systems other than the lungs will generally elicit symptoms related to that organ system and can also manifest as nonspecific ones such as fatigue. The difficulty is that TB is often not the first diagnosis the clinician may consider, leading to delay in treatment. For example, in symptoms of TB of the bowel, particularly in the United States and Western Europe, Crohn disease or cancer would be considered first (Bruckstein, 1988). Thus, in extrapulmonary TB, as in pulmonary TB, a high index of suspicion is useful in making a prompt diagnosis (Elder, 1992). As discussed in Chapter 3, extrapulmonary TB is more common in those who are HIV-infected, in foreign-born persons, and in racial and ethnic minorities

(Felton & Ford, 1993). Major extrapulmonary sites and their specific signs and symptoms of infection are listed in Table 4.1.

Presentation of TB in HIV Infection

Reactivation of a past, latent TB infection often occurs early in HIV infection and may be a presenting condition. Thus, it has been recommended that testing for HIV should accompany the diagnosis of TB (Barnes, Le, & Davidson, 1993; Pitchenik & Fertel, 1992). Likewise, any person with HIV infection should be evaluated for TB (DiFerdinando, Glassroth, Hecht, & Stover, 1993). The presentation of TB may be atypical, particularly in those HIV-infected persons with greater immunosuppression (Haas & Des Prez, 1994). The non-specific symptoms of TB such as malaise, weight loss, and night sweats are also those seen as part of HIV disease, and so an index of suspicion for TB is necessary. Thoracic lymphadenopathy may be seen. Chest radiographs may be atypical and include diffuse pulmonary infiltrates and may be related to immune depression as reflected by the CD4+ count. In one series in those who were not severely immunosuppressed, cavitation and pulmonary effusion were seen more commonly, whereas in those who were severely immunosuppressed, hilar adenopathy and a miliary pattern were seen more often. In addition, extrapulmonary involvement is frequent and is inversely related to the CD4+ count. The extrapulmonary types most frequently seen are lymphadenitis, bacteremia, intra-abdominal disease, and central nervous system disease, particularly meningitis. (Barnes, et al., 1993).

Testing and Diagnosis

If the clinician suspects tuberculosis on the basis of clinical presentation, the next step is generally obtaining a history of possible exposure. For example, if the patient gives a history of working in a prison with an inmate recently placed on treatment for TB, this could mean recent exposure for that patient. Obtaining information about exposure also helps to identify other contacts who will need follow-up as described in Chapter 10.

The history of past tuberculin skin test results compared to current results can help to determine if the onset of disease may be due to reactivation of an old tuberculous infection to the disease state, or whether it reflects recently acquired exogenous disease. The tuberculin skin test can be reactive in both infection and disease, and does not distinguish between them. Further, skin tests may be falsely negative because of anergy or for other reasons. Thus, a reactive tuberculin skin test supports the notion that the patient problem being evaluated may be TB, but a negative skin test does not rule out that possibility. See Chapter 8 for a discussion of tuberculin skin testing.

The next step in assessment is the chest radiograph (x-ray). The patient presenting with symptoms strongly suggestive of TB, regardless of the skin test results, should have a chest x-ray. If extrapulmonary disease is suspected, then studies aimed at the organ system believed to be involved should be undertaken as well. For example, if renal TB is suspected, an intravenous pyelogram might be done (Mandell, Douglas, & Bennett, 1990).

For pulmonary TB, sputum is generally collected for detection of acid-fast bacilli (AFB) in a smear. However, the "gold standard" of diagnosis is culture, which allows the species to be identified and drug susceptibility testing to be done. The drawback is that because *M. tuberculosis* grows slowly (See Chapter 2), the results of the culture may not be available for weeks, although with newer techniques this can be shorter (Glassroth, 1993). In *all* cases, the initial isolate should have drug susceptibility studies performed to optimize therapy and check for drug resistant strains.

Diagnosing tuberculosis involves the assessment of signs and symptoms, history of exposure and test results. A presumptive diagnosis of TB and initiation of therapy will usually be made prior to the completion of culture results. This is important from the standpoint of protecting others from contracting infection and to prevent progression of disease within the individual—particularly important in those with HIV-disease, in whom TB can be rapidly progressive and fatal. However, when multi-drug-resistant TB is strongly suspected, and the patient's condition allows it, the clinician may elect to delay treatment until drug susceptibility study results and available.

LABORATORY TESTING AND DIAGNOSIS

In both the community health and outpatient settings, laboratory testing and diagnosis of TB may follow tuberculin skin testing (discussed at length in Chapter 8) in those who have participated in this type of screening program and have been found to be reactive or may follow clinical suspicion. Tests may be direct or indirect. Indirect tests include tuberculin skin testing, chest radiographs and other imaging techniques, and general blood and fluid analysis. Direct tests are often considered confirmatory and include staining for acid-fast bacilli (AFB), culture techniques, direct biopsy, and newer tests such as radiometric assays, nucleic acid probes with or without polymerase chain reaction, chromatography, and others (Glassroth, 1993). The use of restriction fragment length polymorphism (RFLP) or DNA fingerprinting is not used as a diagnostic test, but is being used epidemiologically to illuminate transmission patterns in a community (Salfinger & Morris, 1994: Schluger & Rom, 1994).

Specimen Collecting and Handling

The quality of the specimen produced and the care with which it is handled after collection are major influences on the outcome of the laboratory studies. Laboratory instructions for collection, handling, and transport should be followed carefully. If a patient is unable to produce a spontaneous specimen, it may be possible to induce one by having the patient inhale aerosolized hypertonic saline which will stimulate sputum production. When collecting specimens, special collection areas such as sputum induction booths equipped with negative pressure and externally forced venting should be used. The health care provider should follow protective procedures so that they are not at risk for acquiring TB (see Chapter 9). Bronchial washing, bronchoalveolar lavage, and/or transbronchial biopsy may be ordered for patients whose sputum is inadequate to support a diagnosis of pulmonary tuberculosis. If a bronchoscopy is performed, sputum will be produced by the patient for several days after the procedure. Daily specimens should be collected and examined in addition to the one obtained during the procedure. Early morning gastric aspiration may be of use in children or adults incapable of producing sputum (MacGregor, 1993). After 8 to 10 hours of fasting and before getting out of bed in the morning, 50 cc of gastric fluid are collected. When extrapulmonary tuberculosis is suspected, other specimens may be needed. If urines are required, midstream early morning (first if possible) specimens are best (American Thoracic Society, 1990). Other body fluids and tissues may be obtained by means of invasive procedures if extrapulmonary TB is suspected. The resulting specimens should be sent to the laboratory as quickly as possible in an appropriate container with either no preservatives or with the correct culture medium.

Laboratory Studies

A standard laboratory test is the sputum smear, which will be positive for AFB in about 50% of persons with pulmonary tuberculosis (MacGregor,

1993). Unfortunately, it may also be positive in persons who do not have tuberculosis but whose lungs are colonized by or infected with one or more of the other species of nontuberculous mycobacteria because it is not specific for *M. tuberculosis*. Thus, a positive AFB sputum smear is not diagnostic for pulmonary tuberculosis. Culture of organisms is done whether or not the AFB smear is positive or negative because an AFB positive smear does not allow for differentiation of species of mycobacteria or identification of drug sensitivities, and those with negative smears may show growth of *M. tuberculosis* in culture. If the cultures grown on standard media are positive, growth should appear within 3 to 6 weeks. If there is growth on cultures, additional chemical tests currently taking 2 to 6 additional weeks are required to determine if the organism growing is *M. tuberculosis* or some other species. Subsequent drug susceptibility tests provide information useful for determining appropriate drug therapy (Glassroth, 1993; Witebsky & Conville, 1993).

Acid-Fast (AFB) Bacilli Smears. A relatively rapid presumptive test for TB is staining for AFB in specimen smears. In body fluids other than sputum, there are relatively few AFB present, so a negative smear examination is not usually very meaningful, whereas a positive result is very useful in these fluids (MacGregor, 1993). The specimen collected in pulmonary TB is sputum, and procedures for collection are described here and in Chapter 6. Morning sputum specimens are best because they generally have the highest number of organisms per volume because of overnight accumulation. Usually at least three specimens are obtained. Although 24-hour collection has been used to collect sputum specimens in those who can produce only small amounts of sputum, because of overgrowth of other bacteria during that time frame, some laboratories will not accept 24-hour specimens for mycobacterial culture (Witebsky et al., 1993). It is important to be sure that sputum, and not saliva, is collected. After processing decontamination, centrifugation may be used to better concentrate the specimen. Then smears are made for AFB staining, and media are inoculated for culture; however, smears may be prepared directly from the specimen. The techniques for staining the specimen include traditional carbol-fuchsin-based stains such as Kinyoun and Ziehl-Neelsen and fluorochrome stains such as auramine-rhodamine. The slide with the traditionally stained smear can then be scanned by means of a low-power microscope. A fluorescent microscope is needed for the fluorochrome stains and uses high-power magnification for smear examination. Examination with the traditionally stained smear is reasonably rapid and low cost making it useful for quick assessment, especially in countries with fewer resources. Limitations include its nonspecificity, meaning that other mycobacterial species such as *Mycobacterium kan-*

saii, produce a positive stain as well as some other organisms such as *Nocardia* (Glassroth, 1993; Salfinger et al., 1994; Witebsky et al., 1993). The laboratory usually makes its report based on the number of AFB seen during scanning of the slide that corresponds to ratings that can range from no AFB seen (rated as negative) through more than 500 colonies (confluence, rated as 4+) according to one scale (American Thoracic Society, 1990; Joklik, Willett, Amos, & Wilfert, 1992). Persons with positive sputum smears are generally considered infectious, although persons with negative sputum smears and positive sputum cultures may also be infectious.

***Cultures*.** Culture of material such as sputum, blood, spinal fluid, and urine or other tissue or fluid for tubercle bacilli has traditionally involved placement on media that are egg- potato based (Lowenstein-Jensen) or agar based (Middlebrook 7H10 or 7H11). These are incubated at 37° C for up to 6 weeks or more in an atmosphere of 10% carbon dioxide and 90% air (Kiehn, 1993; Witebsky et al., 1993). After culture, identification of *M. tuberculosis* is based on such components as the morphology of colonies, growth rates, and biochemical assays. Cultures of infected tissue have yields of from 40 to 80% (MacGregor, 1993). Newer systems and methods that give faster results have or are being developed. The NAP (p-nitro-alpha-acetylamino-beta- hydroxypropiophenone) growth inhibition test differentiates *M. tuberculosis* from other mycobacteria in about a week when used with a radiometric system such as BACTEC (Becton Dickinson) that allows the presence of mycobacteria to be detected before visible growth. These methods have shortened the diagnostic time frame. Chromatography can distinguish species of mycobacteria as can DNA probes (Glassroth, 1993; Kiehn, 1993; Roberts & Thompson, 1994; Witebsky et al., 1993).

***Other Tests*.** Direct testing offers the advantage of not having to wait for culture growth but being able to use clinical specimens directly. Sometimes, techniques such as target or signal amplification are used to increase sensitivity. Polymerase chain reaction (PCR) is an example of target amplification (Kiehn, 1993). DNA probes are not currently sensitive enough alone as a direct method, and thus require culturing, meaning that a week or more is necessary for results. However, when perfected, the combination of PCR with DNA probes should have high sensitivity and specificity and be accomplished in days. Other techniques include mass spectroscopy or gas-liquid chromatography (GLC) for tuberculostearic acid (a fatty acid present in mycobacterial cell walls) and immunoassays for mycobacterial antigens and antibodies or for catalases (Cage,

1994; Glassroth, 1993; Kiehn, 1993; Schluger & Rom, 1994; Witebsky et al., 1993).

Chest Radiographs

The chest radiograph or x-ray is one of the most important tools in the diagnosis of TB and may be used for screening in specific high-risk populations and/or as part of the diagnosis of pulmonary TB. Virtually any abnormality may be seen, particularly in the young, the elderly, or in persons with HIV-infection. In those with intact immunity, typical chest radiograph findings of progressive primary TB include air space consolidation in the middle and lower zones and anterior segments of the upper lobes. Pleural effusion, hilar or mediastinal lymphadenopathy, and miliary dissemination, seen as small nodules distrubuted throughout the lungs, may also occur. In postprimary or reactivation TB, consolidation that is patchy and nodular is usually seen in the upper lobes of one or both lungs (Davis, Yankelevitz, Williams, & Henschke, 1993; Hopewell, 1988; Miller & Miller, 1993; Rossman & Mayock, 1994). These shadows occur most often in the apical or subapical posterior segment of the upper lobes or the superior segment of the lower lobe (Centers for Disease Control and Prevention, 1994; Rossman & Mayock, 1994). Cavitation may also be present (Schluger & Rom, 1994) and is found in about 40% of adult cases, and pleural effusion may be seen in about 19% (Miller et al., 1993). Other findings are possible, particularly in the elderly, those with HIV-disease, and those with other diseases such as cancer. In persons with HIV-infection, the pulmonary involvement is often diffuse and is less likely to be apical or cavitary because the person cannot mount an intense inflammatory response. Hilar and mediastinal lymphadenopathy may be seen (Hopewell, 1992; MacGrgor, 1993; Schluger & Rom, 1994). It is possible that a "normal" chest radiograph may be seen in HIV- infected persons with active TB (Glassroth, 1993). Thus, a high index of suspicion is warranted, and the expertise of a physician experienced in both HIV-infection and TB may be necessary.

Other Imaging Techniques

Computed tomography (CT) of the chest may be useful in specific situations to clarify confusing findings but is generally not necessary to diagnose TB. It may reveal pleural effusions, or unsuspected cavitation or miliary disease patterns (Davis, et at., 1993; Glassroth, 1993). Magnetic resonance imaging (MRI) or ultrasound can be useful in identifying organ involvement in patients with extrapulmonary disease but are usually not diagnostic (Glassroth, 1993).

After Testing and Diagnosis

With an index of suspicion of active TB, even while awaiting confirmed diagnosis, drug therapy may be begun. This therapy may need to be adjusted depending upon drug-susceptibility testing results. Preventive therapy and medical and surgical treatments for TB, as well as patient monitoring of therapy, are discussed in Chapter 5. All suspected (and confirmed) cases of active TB should be reported to the local health department. It is important to identify the contacts of patients with active TB in order to prevent spread of disease (See Chapter 10).

SUMMARY

The symptoms of TB are often subtle and nonspecific, particularly in the elderly or those with HIV disease. In extrapulmonary sites, signs and symptoms are likely to be site specific, and diagnosis (particularly in developed countries) is likely to be delayed. The key to the diagnosis of TB is a high index of suspicion, particularly if individuals have characteristics or conditions placing them at high risk. Newer diagnostic techniques hold the promise of earlier definitive diagnosis. Education, appropriate therapy, and the investigation of contacts to contain the spread of TB may precede the confirmation of the diagnosis.

REFERENCES

American Thoracic Society (1990). Diagnostic standards and classification of tuberculosis. *American Review of Respiratory Disease, 142*, 725-735.

American Thoracic Society. (1994). Treatment of tuberculosis and tuberculosis infection in adults and children. *American Journal of Respiratory and Critical Care Medicine, 149*, 1359-1374.

Barnes, P. F., Le, H. Q., & Davidson, P. T. (1993). Tuberculosis in patients with HIV infection. *Medical Clinics of North America, 77(6)*, 1369-1390.

Bruckstein, A. H. (1988). Abdominal tuberculosis. *New York State Journal of Medicine, 88*, 18-21.

Cage, G. D. (1994). Direct identification of *Mycobacterium* species in BAC-TEC 7H12B medium by high-performance liquid chromatography. *Journal of Clinical Microbiology, 32*, 521-524.

Centers for Disease Control. (1994). Guidelines for preventing the transmission of *Mycobacterium tuberculosis* in health-care facilities, 1994. *Morbidity and Mortality Weekly Report, 43* (RR-13), 1-133.

Couser, J. I. Jr., & Glassroth, J. (1993). Tuberculosis: An epidemic in older adults. *Clinics in Chest Medicine, 14(3)*, 491-499.

Crawford, J. T. (1993). Applications of molecular methods to epidemiology of tuberculosis. *Research Microbiology, 144*, 111-116.

Davis, S. D., Yankelevitz, D. F., Williams, T. & Henschke, C. I. (1993). Pulmonary tuberculosis in immunocompromised hosts: epidemiological, clinical, and radiological assessment. *Seminars in Roentgenology, XXVIII*, 119-130.

DiFerdinando, G. T. Jr., Glassroth, J., Hecht, F. M., & Stover, D. E. (1993). TB and HIV: A deadly synergy. *Patient Care, 27(14)*, 92-114.

Elder, N. C. (1992). Extrapulmonary tuberculosis. *Archives of Family Medicine, 1* 91-98.

Felton, C. P. & Ford, J. G. (1993). Tuberculosis in the inner city. *Lung Biology in Health and Disease, 66*, 483-503.

Glassroth, J. (1993). Diagnosis of tuberculosis. *Lung Biology in Health and Disease, 66,* 149-165.

Haas, D. W., & Des Prez, R. M. (1994). Tuberculosis and acquired immunodeficiency syndrome: A historical perspective on recent developments. *American Journal of Medicine, 96*, 439-450.

Hopewell, P.C. (1988). Mycobacterial diseases. In J.F. Murray & J.A. Nadel (Eds.), *Textbook of respiratory medicine* (pp. 856-915). Philadelphia, PA.: W.B. Saunders Co.

Iseman, M. D. (1993). Treatment of multidrug-resistant tuberculosis. *New England Journal of Medicine, 329*, 784-791.

Iseman, M.D.,& Madsen, L.A. (1989). Drug resistant tuberculosis. *Clinics in Chest Medicine. 10 (3)*,341–353.

Joklik, W. K., Willett, H. P., Amos, D. B., & Wilfert, C. M. (1992). *Zinsser microbiology.* (20th ed.). Norwalk, CT: Appleton & Lange.

Kiehn, T. E. (1993). The diagnostic mycobacteriology laboratory of the 1990s. *Clinical Infectious Diseases, 17(suppl2)* S447–454.

MacGregor, R. R. (1993). Tuberculosis: From history to current management. *Seminars in Roentgenology, XXVIII,* 101–108.

Mandell, G. L., Douglas, R. G. Jr., & Bennett, J. (Eds.). (1990). *Principles and Practice of Infectious Diseases.* (3rd ed.). New York: Churchill Livingstone.

Miller, W. T., & Miller, W. T. Jr. (1993). Tuberculosis in the normal host: radiological findings. *Seminars in Roentgenology, XXVIII,* 109–118.

Pitchenik, A. E. & Fertel, D. (1992). Mycobacterial disease in patients with HIV infection. In G. P. Wormser (Ed.)., *AIDS and other manifestations of HIV infection* (2nd ed.) pp. 277–313. New York: Raven Press. Ltd.

Roberts, G. D., & Thompson, G. P. (1994). Bacteriology and bacteriologic diagnosis of tuberculosis. In D. Schlossberg (Ed). *Tuberculosis* (3rd ed.), (pp. 51–61). New York: Springer-Verlag.

Rossman, M. D., Mayock, R. L. (1994). Pulmonary tuberculosis. In D. Schlossberg (Ed). *Tuberculosis* (3rd ed.), (pp. 95–105). New York: Springer-Verlag.

Salfinger, M., & Morris, A. J. (1994). The role of the microbiology laboratory in diagnosing mycobacterial diseases. *American Journal of Clinical Pathology, 101 (Suppl),* S6–S13.

Schluger, N. W., & Rom, W. N. (1994). Current approaches to the diagnosis of active pulmonary tuberculosis. *American Journal of Respiratory and Critical Care Medicine, 149,* 264–267.

Witebsky, F. G., & Conville, P. S. (1993). The laboratory diagnosis of mycobacterial disease. *Infectious Disease Clinics of North America, 7(2),* 359–376.

Wolinsky, E. (1988). Tuberculosis. In Wyngaarden J.B., Smith, L.H., Bennett, J.C. (Eds.). *Cecil textbook of medicine, vol.2.* (19th ed pp. 1733–1742). Philadelphia: W.B. Saunders.

5

MEDICAL TREATMENT OF TUBERCULOSIS

Lorie Madsen and Felissa L. Cohen

In most cases of drug-susceptible TB, cure is achievable if the proper therapy is initiated and the patient completes treatment. If initial treatment fails for any reason, there is a risk of developing drug-resistant organisms. Treatment of drug-resistant disease is difficult and fraught with management problems such as drug side effects and toxicity and the continued contagious state of the patient, which may in turn promote the spread of primary drug-resistant disease to others. The presence of HIV/AIDS means additional complications relating to its unusual presentation and the vulnerability of the patient. This chapter will describe the medical treatment of tuberculosis and the special concerns of those with multidrug-resistant disease and HIV/AIDS.

DRUG TREATMENT PRINCIPLES

Drug therapy has been the most common approach for the treatment of TB, although in some cases (as discussed later in this chapter) surgical

TABLE 5.1 *M. tuberculosis* **Populations and Effective Drugs**

Mycobacteria Population	Most Effective Chemotherapeutic Agents
1) Extracellular rapidly dividing as in the lung	Isoniazid, Streptomycin, Rifampin
2) Intracellular, within caseous foci; are usually dormant with some periods of increased velocity	Rifampin
3) Intracellular mycobacteria within macrophages	Pyrazinamide, Isoniazid, Rifampin

Source: Ebert (1989)

intervention can prove useful. Several drugs have been traditionally used to treat tuberculosis, and new ones have been added to that armamentarium. When making decisions about initial therapy for TB, it is important to evaluate the risk that multidrug-resistant (MDR) tuberculosis may be present. Some risk factors for the presence or development of MDR-TB (either primary or acquired) include prior drug treatment for TB; contact with a person recently treated for TB; the presence of or predisposing factors to HIV infection or immunosuppression; history of close contact with persons with HIV-infection or immunosuppression or predisposing factors to HIV infection; residence in institutions such as jails, hospitals, or shelters in areas with high prevalence of MDR-TB; being an immigrant from a country with a high prevalence of MDR-TB; and residence in a geographic locale with high a prevalence of MDR-TB (Centers for Disease Control, 1992; Wolinsky, 1993).

Typically, TB drug treatment regimens have included several therapeutic agents that have been administered daily over a long period of time. It was not until the 1960s that drug regimen durations were reduced to 18 months from an average of 24 months. In the 1970s short course regimens with durations of 9 months were the treatment standard; adding another drug to the regimen allowed therapy to be shortened to 6 months, with some protocols allowing two to three times a week administration (Ellner, et al., 1993). However, nonadherence has been noted to be a problem even with shortened treatment protocols for various reasons including improvement in symptoms, side effects of medication, and the hassles associated with taking medication every day. It is important that the patient complete the course of therapy because failure to do so can result in the development of drug-resistant strains.

It is thought that, in pulmonary TB, there are bacilli in 3 types of physiologic conditions: 1) rapidly multiplying ones in the well-oxygenated pulmonary cavity extracellular environment; 2) more slowly metabolizing organisms in solid caseous material constituting an acidic environment that is somewhat less oxygenated; and 3) those in an acidic environment within the activated macrophage (intracellular). Treatment is directed, therefore, at both the extracellular and intracellular organisms with an initial bacteriocidal phase and a subsequent sterilizing stage. Therapeutic agents must attack those organisms that are actively growing; those that are dormant with intermittent spurts of activity; and those within an acid environment such as within phagocytes and caseous foci (Ebert, 1989). (see Table 5.1). Combinations of drugs are used in treatment 1) to eliminate extracellular mycobacteria rapidly, thereby decreasing infectivity; and 2) to eliminate mycobacteria within caseous foci or granulomas and within the macrophages. Thus a first or induction phase of therapy is aimed at rapidly killing extracellular mycobacteria with an agent such as isoniazid (INH), and the second or continuation phase is aimed at eliminating persistent organisms ("persisters") by use of sterilizing drugs such as rifampin (RIF) or pyrazinamide (PZA) (Ebert, 1989). In addition, treatment strategy includes a selection of drugs that is made on the basis of the status of TB, site, and the risk of multidrug-resistant TB.

TYPICAL THERAPEUTIC AGENTS USED TO TREAT TUBERCULOSIS

Agents used to treat TB are divided into "firstline" and "secondline" drugs. Firstline agents include isoniazid, rifampin, pyrazinamide, ethambutol, and streptomycin. Secondline agents include cycloserine, ethionamide, kanamycin, para-aminosalicylic acid, and capreomycin. Isoniazid and rifampin have been called essential in the treatment of TB (Ellner et al., 1993). The actions and major features about each drug are discussed below; specific dosage recommendations and other information are given in Table 5.2, whereas treatment combinations and regimens for both adults and children with and without HIV infection are discussed later in this chapter and in Tables 5.4 and 5.5.

First-Line Agents

Isoniazid (INH)(Laniazid, Teebaconin) is the most widely used drug against TB and is called the keystone of TB therapy (Mandell, Douglas,

(continued, p. 74)

TABLE 5.2 Selected Information About the Most Common Drugs Used to Treat Tuberculosis*

Drug/Dose/ Administration	Side Effects/Toxicity	Comments
ISONIAZID 5mg/kg up to 300 mg po daily; Can be given IM.	Hepatitis, peripheral neuropathy that is usually dose related. Nausea, vomiting, fatigue anorexia, malaise, weakness, epigastric distress are possible. Rare CNS effects, lupus syndrome. Hypersensitivity. Elevations of serum hepatic transaminases and bilirubin with phenytoin (Dilantin).	B_6 (pyridoxine) with each dose may decrease peripheral neuropathy and CNS effects. Evaluate phenytoin levels in patients with seizures. Monitor serum transaminases. Have patient report numbness or tingling in hands or feet. Teach patient to report symptoms of liver damage (dark urine, jaundice; nausea, vomiting, unexplained anorexia, unexplained fatigue, fever and/or abdominal tenderness.)
RIFAMPIN (Rifadin, Rimactane) 600 mg po daily, 450 mg if <50 kg wt. IV form available.	GI effects such as nausea, vomiting, heartburn, epigastric distress, jaundice, cramps, and diarrhea. Skin reactions such as pruritus, flushing with or without a rash. Colors body fluids (e.g. urine, saliva, sweat, sputum, tears) orange. Many drug interactions—increases anticoagulant (such as Coumadin) requirements; diminishes methadone effectiveness; alters oral contraceptive effectiveness; reduces activity of other drugs such as corticosteroids, cyclosporine,	Administer in single doses, on an *empty* stomach (2 hrs before or after meals). Warn patients to expect orange coloration of body secretions. Discuss other medications patient is taking and be alert for need for adjustment of medications. Counsel patient on other forms of birth control if taking oral contraceptives. If taking with old PAS preparations, take at least 8 hours apart because rifampin blood levels

70

Table 5.2, continued

Drug/Dose/Administration	Side Effects/Toxicity	Comments
	oral hypoglycemic agents, dapsone, analgesics, quinidine, ketoconazole, theophylline, and cardiac glycoside preparations. Hepatitis, thrombocytopenia may occur, flulike syndrome (chills, malaise, headache, pain, fever) with intermittent rather than daily administration.	may otherwise decrease. Diabetes may be more difficult to control. Monitor transaminase blood levels for liver function. Patients who use methadone may need increased dose.
ETHAMBUTOL (Myambutol) 15-25 mg/kg po daily	Optic neuritis, with blurred vision, central scotomata and red-green color blindness. GI discomfort, pruritus, confusion, joint pain, rash, fever, tingling, and numbness of extremities. Increased uric acid in blood.	Check visual acuity (with Snellen chart)/color vision monthly. Advise patient to report changes in visual acuity, or red-green color discrimination changes which can be unilateral or bilateral such as blurred vision.
PYRAZINAMIDE 30 mg/kg po daily	Contraindicated in severe hepatic damage and acute gout. Caution in those with diabetes mellitus because it can interfere with management. May experience mild arthralgia or myalgia. Elevated uric acid, hepatotoxicity, GI discomfort.	Treat uric acid elevation if symptomatic. Start with divided daily doses and consolidate. Monitor liver function, especially SGOT and uric acid levels, monthly. Teach patient to notify if fever, anorexia, malaise, nausea and vomiting, dark urine, jaundice, pain or swelling of joints are present.
STREPTOMYCIN 15mg/kg up to 1g/day initially or 25-30mg/kg up to 1.5g/d in twice-a-week regimens IM.	Ototoxicity; can cause eighth cranial nerve damage. Nausea, vomiting, vertigo, hearing loss. May feel numbness around mouth or giddiness. Caution in renal insufficiency and elderly; may see minor tubular dysfunction.	Baseline and periodic (usually monthly) audiometric and vestibular testing. Have patient report hearing problems and/or dizziness. Ultrasound and/or hot packs to injection site. Monitor serum BUN and creatinine levels.

Drug/Dose/ Administration	Side Effects/Toxicity	Comments
KANAMYCIN 15–30mg/kg to maximum dose of 1g/day IM or IV.	Nephrotoxicity, ototoxicity (affects eighth cranial nerve); can cause hearing loss, neuromuscular blockade.	As in streptomycin. Auditory dysfunction more common than vestibular. Keep patient well-hydrated.
ETHIONAMIDE (Trecator-SC) 500–1000 mg daily po, usually divided doses.	GI intolerance, including anorexia, nausea, vomiting, abdominal pain, and a metallic taste. Depression, headache, drowsiness, psychological distrubances. Rarely are gynecomastia, impotence, hair loss, menstrual irregularities seen; hypothyroidism; hepatotoxicity and hepatitis; difficulties in management of diabetes. Arthralgias and dermatitis may occur.	Monitor serum transaminase. Take with food. Antacids, antiemetics help tolerance. Start with 250 mg and increase dose gradually. Counsel patients about possible side effects. Watch for difficulty in managing diabetic patients. Hypothyroidism is *very* common if used in conjunction with PAS.
CYCLOSERINE (Seromycin) 250–1000 mg. daily po, usually divided doses.	Nervous system and psychiatric effects: forgetfulness, confusion, behavior changes, peripheral neuropathy, depression, headache, psychosis, seizures, tremors, somnolence, vertigo, paresis, dysarthria. May be contraindicated in epilepsy, pre-existing depression, anxiety or psychiatric disorders, severe renal insufficiency, or excessive concurrent use of alcohol. Rash.	Introduce gradually. Start with 250 mg and check serum levels; doses are increased until stable. Aim for peak serum concentrations between 10–35 mcg/ml for best effects without toxicity. Anticonvulsants may be used to control CNS effects such as seizures. Can give pyridoxine with each dose to try to prevent toxicity. Mental status should be assessed regularly. Patients and families should be alerted to report difficulty in speaking, personality changes, twitching, dizziness, forgetfulness, or memory loss as well as other symptoms and can be taught to write things down, make lists etc. Alcohol should be avoided.

Table 5.2, continued

Drug/Dose/ Administration	Side Effects/Toxicity	Comments
PARA- AMINOSALICYLIC ACID (Teebacin) 150 mg/kg to 10–12 gm po daily, usually divided doses. New preparation is sustained release granules (Paser) in 4 gm packets without sodium.	High frequency of gastrointestinal effects such as epigastric discomfort, nausea, vomiting, diarrhea, cramps, anorexia. Fever, malaise, joint pains, rash, or sore throat may occur. Hypothyroidism may occur.	Begin with 1–2 gms. tid or qid and increase as tolerated over a few days. Give with acidic drink or food or after meals. Use antacids and antiemetics for GI distress. Monitor cardiac patients due to sodium load if using older tablet preparation. Be alert for nonadherence because of GI distress. Hypothyroidism is common if used in conjunction with ethionamide.
CAPREOMYCIN Usual dose is 20 mg/kg per day not to exceed 1 gm, IM. IV form available.	May be contraindicated in those with audiometric impairment or renal insufficiency. Weigh against benefits. Affects eighth cranial nerve. Dizziness, high tone acuity loss and other hearing loss, vertigo; renal insufficiency.	Assess audiometric and vestibular function before beginning therapy and at monthly intervals. Teach patient to report hearing problems, dizziness, balance problems; monitor BUN and creatinine. Should not be used with other ototoxic or nephrotoxic drugs.
CIPROFLOXACIN (Cipro) 500–750 mg daily po	Gastrointestinal symptoms, such as abdominal pain, nausea, vomiting, diarrhea. Headache, restlessness, rash, dizziness. May increase serum levels of Coumadin® , theophylline, and caffeine. Interaction with probenecid. May cause photosensitivity. Hypersensitivity reaction.	Preferably take 2 hours after meals. Drink fluids liberally. Avoid products with iron or zinc (such as multivitamins), sucralfate, and antacids with magnesium, aluminum, or calcium. May need to adjust medications in patients using theophylline or on

Table 5.2, continued

Drug/Dose/Administration	Side Effects/Toxicity	Comments
		anticoagulants. Limit caffeine if insomnia or restlessness occur. Advise about possible dizziness or light-headedness for operating car or machinery. Avoid direct sunlight (use sunscreen).
OFLOXACIN (Floxacin) 400–800 mg daily po	Hypersensitivity. GI distress including nausea, diarrhea, vomiting, abdominal pain, anorexia. Headache, insomnia, dizziness, vaginitis, and vaginal pruritis in women, rash. Phototoxicity. May increase serum levels of Coumadin®, theophylline.	As above for ciprofloxacin.

*Any of these drugs can cause hypersensitivity reactions. Not all side effects/toxicities are listed. Doses of some of the medications listed may be different in treating drug resistant infection or disease. The elderly, those with HIV infection, and children may require special considerations.

& Bennett, 1990). It is a potent bacteriocidal agent, acting by inhibiting synthesis of a major component of the cell wall of *M. tuberculosis*. It kills rapidly growing mycobacteria extracellularly and inhibits growth of mycobacteria that may be dormant within the macrophages and in caseous lesions (Ebert, 1989). Its small molecular size means that it is distributed widely, penetrating into body fluids and tissues, including caseous lesions, phagocytic cells, amniotic fluid, breast milk and cerebrospinal fluid (Brausch & Bass, 1993; Mandell, et al., 1990; O'Brien, 1993). It is administered orally, although an injectable version is now available for limited use. It is metabolized by the liver. Hepatitis is a major toxic effect (American Thoracic Society, 1994; O'Brien, 1993). It is estimated that clinical hepatitis develops in 1% to 2% of all patients taking INH and as many as 10% to 20% develop elevations of hepatic enzymes and/or bilirubin (Brausch et al., 1993). This hepatitis is age-related with the risk increasing in persons over 35 years of age. Persons who have the genetically determined metabolizing trait of rapid acetylators are more likely to develop such problems than those who are slow acetylators. Because INH depletes pyridoxine stores, those with conditions resulting in deficiency of pyridoxine (e.g., pregnancy, diabetes, uremia, alcoholism, malnutrition, cancer), and those with seizures usually need daily supplementation in order to prevent peripheral neuropathy (occurring in a "stocking-glove" distribution) which is a second major toxic effect (Mandell, et al., 1990; O'Brien, 1993). Persons taking phenytoin (Dilantin) may need the dosage adjusted (Physicians' Desk Reference, 1994).

Rifampin (RIF, RMP) (Rifadin, Rimactane) is the second major anti-TB agent and is a semisynthetic antibiotic derivative of rifamycin B (Physicians' Desk Reference, 1994). It can be administered orally or intravenously. It is also bacteriocidal, inhibiting DNA-dependent RNA polymerase (an essential enzyme) in *M. tuberculosis* (Mandell & Sande, 1990). Rifampin penetrates well into tissues and cells including caseous lesions, phagocytic cells, and inflamed meninges. There is some question about how well it penetrates into noninflamed meninges. RIF is also metabolized by the liver, inducing hepatic microsomal enzymes, and therefore also may accelerate clearance of other drugs and hormones such as Coumadin® , methadone, oral contraceptive agents, antiarrhythmic drugs (e.g., quinidine, mexiletine HCl, and verapamil), theophylline, anticonvulsants, ketoconazole, and others, making them less effective. Thus, those in methadone maintenance programs may legitimately require increased dosages. Persons with disease conditions such as asthma who are taking theophylline will need medication adjustment. Because of the effect on oral contraceptives, birth control alternatives need to be discussed with females of reproductive age. Skin reactions such as pruritus and flushing with or without a rash, and gastrointestinal effects such as heartburn, anorexia, nausea, vomiting, cramps, and diarrhea have been noted. Hepatitis is a major toxic effect; thus, careful assessment is necessary to design appropriate drug therapy for those taking multiple therapeutic agents to ensure effectiveness and prevent complications. Another untoward effect of rifampin is its reddish orange discoloration of body fluids such as urine, tears, saliva, semen, sweat, and feces. This effect can result in permanent discoloration of soft contact lenses. Persons taking rifampin should be advised about this body fluid discoloration (Brausch & Bass, 1993; O'Brien, 1993). A combination capsule of INH and RIF (Rifamate; Marion Merrell Dow) is available (Barnes, Le et al., 1993).

Pyrazinamide (PZA). This is a nicotinic acid derivative that is bacteriocidal in an acid environment and is particularly active against *M. tuberculosis* intracellularly such as within macrophages, and at the center of caseous foci, although the exact mechanism of action is unknown. It penetrates most tissues and enters the cerebrospinal fluid. Because it is metabolized to a product that competes with uric acid for renal secretion, hyperuricemia often occurs with some joint pain. Caution is needed in those with diabetes mellitus because it interferes with management. Hepatotoxicity is also seen, and both uric acid levels and liver function should be closely monitored. Patients should be observed for and/or report jaundice, fever, anorexia, nausea and vomiting, dark urine, joint swelling and pain. A combination tablet of INH, RIF, and PZA (Rifaten) is now available (Mandell, et al., 1990; O'Brien, 1993; Physicians' Desk Reference, 1994).

Ethambutol (EMB) (Myambutol). At usual doses, ethambutol is bacteriostatic against *M. tuberculosis*, with bacteriocidal effects at higher dosages. It appears to inhibit mycobacterial RNA synthesis. It does not penetrate well into cerebrospinal fluid. The most serious side effect is optic neuritis (retrobulbar) that is evidenced by symptoms as central scotomata, decreased red-green color vision, blurred vision, and sometimes gun-barrel vision. Patients should be educated to let the health care professional know if visual changes occur. A patient on EMB should have periodic assessment of at least a Snellen eye exam and color vision assessment. Symptoms of toxicity may be subtle, such as a complaint of mild blurring noticed during reading, or when watching TV. Occasionally, the patient will notice and report difficulty distinguishing colors, particularly red-green discrimination. The drug should be stopped and a formal ophthalmologic examination performed. Often, some, if not all, of the visual changes may clear but recovery can be slow, as long as a year. Ocular effects are more commonly seen in patients with renal insufficiency. Because of the difficulty in testing young children for the visual effects, ethambutol is not usually a drug of choice for young children (American Thoracic Society, 1994; et al., Ebert, 1989; Mandell, 1990; O'Brien, 1993).

Streptomycin. (SM) Streptomycin is an aminoglycoside antibiotic that is bacteriocidal at neutral or alkaline pHs, and is useful extracellularly. It is given parentally, and excretion is mainly renal (O'Brien, 1993). For many years streptomycin was hard to obtain in the United States, but became available in May 1993 (Di Ferdinando, Glassroth, Hecht, & Stover, 1993). A major side effect is damage to the eighth cranial nerve (the acoustic nerve with cochlear and vestibular branches) causing ototoxicity. The damage results in vestibular dysfunction including nausea, vomiting, and vertigo as well as hearing loss (Brausch & Bass, 1993; Peloquin, 1993). Some clinicians recommend baseline vestibular and audiometric testing with periodic repeats to monitor hearing and vestibular function (Ebert, 1989). Hearing loss usually begins in the high frequencies and progresses toward the speech range; thus audiometric testing will detect loss before it is perceived by the patient. If vestibular toxicity occurs, the drug may need to be discontinued. It is important to monitor and question the patient for possible dizziness or balance problems, and assessment can include the Romberg test, heel-to-toe walking, and a quick turn while walking (Brausch et al., 1993; O'Brien, 1993; Perez-Stable & Hopewell, 1989). Vestibular toxicity is serious and may be permanent. Streptomycin should be used cautiously or avoided in the elderly because of its ototoxic and nephrotoxic effects (American Thoracic Society, 1994). It can be toxic to the fetus.

Second-Line Agents

Cycloserine (Seromycin) is a broad-spectrum antibiotic that is bacteriostatic, acting by inhibiting mycobacterial cell wall synthesis. It is is used mainly for MDR-TB, is administered orally and penetrates well into most body tissues and fluids including cerebrospinal fluid. It is excreted renally. Its major side effects are dose-related central nervous system and psychiatric problems, such as headache, impaired cognition, nervousness, seizures, peripheral neuropathy (especially when given with INH), depression, aggravation of previous psychiatric illnesses, and vertigo. These are more common in alcoholic patients. Pyridoxine may be given with cycloserine in an attempt to prevent neurologic toxicity (Ebert, 1989; Iseman, 1993; Peloquin, 1993). Counseling the patient to expect some memory loss is extremely important. They may need to get in the habit of writing down ideas and making lists while on therapy with this drug. Reaction times may be delayed which can have implications for driving a car or operating machinery. A reliable person may need to evaluate the patient's ability to perform tasks safely. Periodic mental status assessment is needed. Patients taking phenytoin may need a dosage reduction of phenytoin (American Thoracic Society, 1994).

Ethionamide (ETA) (Trecator-SC) is an oral bacteriostatic agent against *M. tuberculosis* and is also used for MDR-TB. Its major adverse effect is gastrointestinal toxicity such as nausea, vomiting, a bitter metallic taste and abdominal pain. It is poorly tolerated and generally used only when necessary (Iseman, 1993). To avoid the poor tolerance, rectal administration has been tried experimentally (Peloquin, 1993) or an antiemetic may be administed about 30 minutes before the cycloserine (American Thoracic Society, 1994). Ethionamide-induced hepatotoxicity takes weeks to resolve once the medication is stopped, and in fact, liver enzymes may continue to rise for a few days despite discontinuing the drug. Hypothyroidism may occur, particularly if the regimen contains PAS, and baseline thyroid testing should be considered before therapy is begun. ETA can rarely cause side effects such as impotence, decreased libido, menstrual irregularity, gynecomastia, hair loss, and joint pain.

Capreomycin (Capastat sulfate) is a polypeptide antibiotic that is bacteriostatic and inhibits mycobacterial protein synthesis. It is given parentally and is excreted renally. Nephrotoxicity is the most common side effect followed by effects on the eighth cranial nerve leading to ototoxicity, vestibular dysfunction, and hearing loss (Ebert; 1989; Mandell, et al., 1990; O'Brien, 1993). Patients should be regularly assessed for proper vestibular function. Older persons are more susceptible to the toxic effects (American Thoracic Society, 1994).

Para-aminosalicylic acid (PAS) was used years ago for TB, often with INH, and has now been mostly replaced in regimens by ethambutol. It is bacteriostatic, given orally, and has frequent gastrointestinal effects (epigastric pain, cramps, nausea, vomiting, diarrhea), and hypersensitivity reactions, as well as some hepatotoxicity. The frequent side effects (as high as 30%) contributed to poor patient compliance (Brausch et al., 1993; Ebert, 1989; Mandell et al., 1990). To prevent gastrointestinal effects, sometimes the person is started on low doses, which are gradually increased to therapeutic levels within a few days. Giving PAS with food reduces local gastric irritation. Antacids and antiemetics or drugs that empty the stomach such as Reglan (metaclopramide) can be extremely helpful, particularly if given approximately one-half hour prior to the drug dose. Gastrointestinal effects of both drugs often limit the use of both ethionamide and PAS at the same time (American Thoracic Society, 1994; Iseman, 1993). The newer preparation of extended release granules does not create a sodium load. It can be taken with acidic food or drink, such as orange juice.

Kanamycin and Amikacin are aminoglycoside antibiotics that have adverse effects such as nephrotoxicity, ototoxicity, and neuromuscular blockade with respiratory paralysis. Interaction with certain diuretics (e.g., furosemide) is common. They are administered intramuscularly or intravenously. Hypersensitivity reactions can occur (Brausch et al., 1993; Physicians' Desk Reference, 1994). Patients should also be monitored for imbalances of calcium, potassium, and magnesium (American Thoracic Society, 1994).

Other Drugs

The fluoroquinalone antibiotics ciprofloxacin (Cipro) and ofloxacin (Floxin) have been used in the treatment of multidrug-resistant TB and other mycobacterial infections. Data on clinical efficacy have been suggestive for retreatment regimens, and these drugs appear to have a place in the successful treatment of MDR-TB. Side effects and toxicity are uncommon, but may include hepatotoxicity, dizziness, nephrotoxicity, insomnia, candidiasis, anxiety, and gastrointestinal symptoms (Brausch et al., 1993; Iseman, 1993; Madsen & Berning, 1993). As of July 1994, these were not licensed for TB treatment in the U.S. (American Thoracic Society, 1994).

Clofazimine (Lamprene) (CF) has been used in the treatment of leprosy, being slowly bacteriocidal against *Mycobacterium leprae* and is being tried in drug-resistant TB, but clinical efficacy is unclear at this time; it may be employed in desperate regimens. Given orally, the usual dose is 100 to 300 mg. per day orally. A major effect is discoloration that is pink-red to brown-black involving the skin, tears, conjunctiva, sweat, urine, and feces that affect 75 to 100% of patients and is a major factor in non-adherence and in feelings of depression in patients. Patient education should include warning of this. Abdominal symptoms and severe pain are also common affecting 40 to 50% of patients, and organ damage can result from crystal deposits. Caution is needed in administration to patients with pre-existing GI problems. Patients should be instructed to take the drug with meals. Skin changes including dryness and pruritis commonly occur. Most patients become a bronze color, which slowly fades once the drug is discontinued; however, exposure to the sun can rapidly potentiate the color change and should be avoided. (American Thoracic Society, 1994; Physicians' Desk Reference, 1994).

Amithiozone and thiacetazone have been used in developing countries because of low cost but are not currently approved by the FDA. They are oral medications with tuberculostatic activity. Side effects are seen more in patients with HIV infection, and thiacetazone may be contraindicated in this group. Side effects include nausea, vomiting, rash, and the Stevens-Johnson syndrome (American Thoracic Society, 1994; Iseman, 1993; O'Brien, 1993).

Clarithromycin (Blaxin) and azithromycin (Zithromax) are macrolide antibiotics that are generally well tolerated, used orally and are being tested for efficacy against *M. tuberculosis* (Ballow, Chapman & Martin, 1993; Brausch et al., 1993). Combinations of clavulanic acid and beta-lactam antibiotics (e.g. amoxicillin-clavulanate) and newer rifamycin antibiotics such as rifambutin, have also been of interest (Iseman, 1993; O'Brien, 1993). New anti-TB drugs are being identified and developed, including the 5-nitroimidazole CGI 17341 and the oxazolidinone DuP 721. New drug delivery systems for anti-TB drugs, such as implantable devices or liposomes, are under investigation (Peloquin & Berning, 1994).

TABLE 5.3 High Priority Candidates for Tuberculosis Preventive Therapy

---

Preventive therapy should be recommended for the following persons with a positive tuberculin test, regardless of age[a]:

- Persons with known or suspected HIV infection.[b]
- Close contacts of persons with infectious clinically active TB.[b]
- Recent tuberculin skin test converters ($\geq$10 mm increase within a 2-year period for those <35 years old; $\geq$15 mm increase for those $\geq$35 years old). All children <4 years with $\geq$10 mm skin test are included in this category.
- Persons with medical conditions that have been reported to increase the risk of TB (e.g. diabetes mellitus, prolonged corticosteroid therapy, immunosuppressive therapy, some hematologic and reticuloendothelial diseases, injecting drug use, end-stage renal disease, and clinical situations associated with rapid weight loss).

Preventive therapy should be recommended for the following persons in high-incidence groups with a tuberculin test $\geq$10 mm who are <35 years old even without additional risk factors.[c]

- Non-U.S.-born persons from high-prevalance countries (e.g. countries in Latin America, Asia, and Africa.
- Medically underserved low-income populations, including high-risk racial or ethnic populations, especially black, Hispanic, and Native American groups.
- Residents of facilities for long-term care) e.g., correctional institutions, nursing homes, and mental institutions).

---

[a]Persons with fibrotic infiltrates on chest radiograph thought to represent old, healed TB and those with silicosis, who were formerly considered candidates for preventive therapy, should receive 4-month multidrug chemotherapy.

[b]Persons in these categories may be given preventive therapy in the absence of a positive tuberculin test in some circumstances.

[c]Staff of facilities in which an individual with current TB would pose a risk to large numbers of susceptible persons (e.g. correctional institutions, nursing homes, mental institutions, other healthcare facilities, schools, and child-care facilities, may also be considered for preventive therapy if their tuberculin reaction is $\geq$10 mm.

Sources: American Thoracic Society (1992). Control of tuberculosis in the United States. *American Review of Respiratory Disease*, *146*, 1629.
American Thoracic Society (1994). Treatment of tuberculosis and tuberculosis infection in adults and children. *American Journal of Respiratory and Critical Care Medicine*, *149*, 1359–1374.

PREVENTIVE CHEMOTHERAPY

As discussed in Chapter 8, a positive Mantoux skin test with normal x-ray findings and no recovery of organisms usually indicates that the individual has tuberculous infection rather than tuberculosis. Preventive drug therapy may be initiated to prevent latent infection from progressing to active disease (secondary prevention) (American Thoracic Society, 1990; American Thoracic Society, 1992, 1994; Mandell et al., 1990). Sometimes, preventive chemotherapy may be initiated for contacts of known active TB cases, especially if close exposure occurred within the past 3 months in order to prevent tuberculous infection from becoming established. This prophylaxis is particularly important for those at high risk for developing tuberculosis clinically after becoming infected and also for children under 4 to 5 years of age (American Thoracic Society, 1990; American Thoracic Society, 1994; Mandell et al., 1990; Miller, 1993). It is important to exclude clinical TB before beginning preventive therapy (Centers for Disease Control and Prevention, 1992). Persons with positive Mantoux tests who are high-priority candidates for preventive therapy are listed in Table 5.3. Preventive therapy in pregnancy should be evaluated on a case-to-case basis (Centers for Disease Control and Prevention, 1994).

Recommended Regimen for Preventive Therapy

The most common drug used for preventive therapy in drug-susceptible TB is isoniazid (INH). For adults, the typical dose is 300 mg daily, and in children, it is 10 to 15 milligrams per kilogram of body weight per day (not exceeding 300 mg). For most adults, 6 continuous months of therapy are recommended; 9 months are recommended for children. For those who are immunosuppressed, such as in HIV infection, 12 months of preventive therapy are recommended (American Thoracic Society, 1992, 1994; Miller, 1993). Persons who have chest radiographs reflecting past TB should also receive 12 months of preventive therapy. If it is suspected that the person may have been infected with an INH-resistant strain of tubercle bacilli, then rifampin (up to 600 milligrams for adults and 10 milligrams per kilogram for children per day, not exceeding 600 milligrams) may be given for 6 to 12 months. Rifampin-pyrazinamide regimens are being investigated to avoid isoniazid toxicity or in cases of INH resistance (Geiter, 1993).

For those who are at risk of developing MDR-TB (e.g., contacts of MDR-TB cases), preventive therapy should be initiated with at least two drugs to which sensitivity has been demonstrated. Because resistance often develops to isoniazid and rifampin, preventive regimens may include combinations such as ethambutol and pyrazinamide or pyrazinamide and ciprofloxacin or ofloxacin (Geiter, 1993). Other regimens for those infected with MDR-TB strains have been suggested and may include ethambutol, pyrazinamide, or a quinolone in various combinations (Miller, 1993).

Preventive therapy is highly effective. In one study, a 6-month course of therapy was 69% effective among those adherent to therapy, and in another study, on a 12-month course of therapy, effectiveness among those who were adherent was 93% (American Thoracic Society, 1992). Preventive therapy regimens in which INH is given at higher dosages on a twice-weekly schedule are being tried for less adherent patients and for those in whom daily therapy cannot be accomplished. The effectiveness of this approach is only suggestive at this time (Miller, 1993).

The American Thoracic Society (1994) has recommended that various evaluations take place before a person starts INH preventive therapy. Every person with a significant tuberculin skin test reaction should have a chest radiograph, and depending on the results, further evaluation to exclude progressive disease. Evaluations before beginning preventive therapy include:

- Exclusion of persons with bacteriologically positive or progressive TB (they need appropriate therapy);
- Determination of any history of previous or current preventive therapy or treatment for TB;
- Assessment of any possible contraindications to INH for preventive therapy such as previous INH-associated hepatic injury, history of severe reactions to INH, and the presence of any acute or unstable liver disease; and
- Identification of persons in whom special precautions may be indicated such as those more than 35 years of age; use of a long-term medication that may interact with INH; daily use of alcohol; history of previous discontinuation of INH; current chronic liver disease; peripheral neuropathy or a condition predisposing to peripheral neuropathy (e.g. diabetes mellitus); injection drug use; post pubertal African-American and Hispanic women, especially postpartum; and pregnancy (American Thoracic Society, 1994).

Prior to embarking on preventive therapy, the patient should be educated about why isoniazid preventive therapy has been prescribed. The signs and symptoms of INH toxicity (as discussed elsewhere in this chapter) should be integral to that education. Baseline liver function tests should be obtained prior to treatment and rechecked periodically. Patients should be monitored monthly to assess adherence to therapy and for possible side effects or toxicity. Persons who are over 35 years of age; those with chronic liver disease; those with a history of hepatic disease, peripheral neuropathy, injecting, or other drug use including alcohol; pregnant women and others at high risk of INH toxicity should be monitored particularly closely (Miller, 1993). Some studies have suggested that black and Hispanic women, particularly postpartum, may be at higher risk for INH-related hepatic toxicity (Geiter, 1993; Snider & Caras, 1992). If signs or symptoms of toxicity occur, discontinuation of INH may be necessary. The American Thoracic Society states that INH preventive therapy should not be given if monthly monitoring cannot be accomplished (1992). For populations with special problems such as alcohol use, any general symptoms such as nausea and vomiting should be evaluated to see if their cause is really INH toxicity before therapy is discontinued.

Preventive therapy is not used as effectively in the United States as it might be. Adherence to preventive therapy is even more difficult than it is for TB treatment when symptoms are present and the person perceives that he or she is ill. Maintaining adherence is important for both the patient and provider. In addition, some believe that because of the risks associated with INH in older people, preventive therapy should be limited to those who are younger (for example under age 35 years) or only to older people who are actually infected rather than noninfected contacts (Miller, 1993). However, others perceive that the preventive benefits outweigh the risk of hepatitis for tuberculin reactors who are at high risk for TB (Geiter, 1993).

DRUG THERAPY FOR INITIAL TUBERCULOSIS TREATMENT

The Centers for Disease Control and Prevention updated their recommendations for the initial therapy of TB in 1993. One of the major reasons for this update was the increasing prevalence of drug-resistant TB in the United States (Centers for Disease Control and Prevention, 1993). The mechanism of occurrence and prevalence of multidrug-resistant TB was discussed in Chapter 3 and later in this chapter. Beginning a patient on a single drug regimen or adding a single drug to a failing regimen or more than 1 month after the start of the primary regimen can lead to the development of mycobacterial populations that are resistant to that drug. Therefore, it is necessary to use a regimen that contains more than one drug to which *M. tuberculosis* is susceptible. In that manner, the emergence of tubercle bacilli that are resistant to one drug will most likely be susceptible to one of the other drugs in the regimen. The vast majority of patients with drug-sensitive TB who adhere to their treatment regimen will achieve cure with proper medical treatment.

The following are the recommended approaches in treatment as detailed by the CDC (1993a):

- Perform drug susceptibility testing on the first isolate of *M. tuber-*

TABLE 5.4 Regimen Options for the Treatment of Tuberculosis (TB) in Children and Adults

Option	Indication	Total Duration of Therapy	Initial Treatment Phase		Continuation Treatment Phase		Comments
			Drugs*	Interval and duration	Drugs*	Interval and duration	
1	Pulmonary and extrapulmonary TB in adults and children	6 mos	INH RIF PZA EMB or SM	Daily for 8 wks	INH RIF	Daily or two or three times wkly+ for 16 wks§	•EMB or SM should be continued until susceptibility to INH and RIF is demonstrated. •In areas where primary INH resistance is <4%, EMB or SM may not be necessary for patients with no individual risk factors for drug resistance.
2	Pulmonary and extrapulmonary TB in adults and children	6mos	INH RIF PZA EMB or SM	Daily for 2 wks, then Two times wkly+ for 6 wks	INH RIF	Two times wkly+ for 16 wks§	•Regimen should be directly observed. •After the initial phase, EMB or SM should be continued until susceptibility to INH and RIF is demonstrated, unless drug resistance is unlikely.
3	Pulmonary and extrapulmonary TB in adults and children	6 mos	INH RIF PZA EMB or SM	3 times wkly+ for 6 mos§			•Regimen should be directly observed. •Continue all four drugs for 6 mos.¶ •This regimen has been shown to be effective for INH-resistant TB.
4	Smear- and culture-negative pulmonary TB in adults	4 mos	INH RIF EMB or SM	Follow option 1, 2, or 3 for 8 wks	INH RIF PZA EMB or SM	Daily or two or three times wkly+ for 8 wks	•Continue all four drugs for 4 mos. •If drug resistance is unlikely (primary INH resistance <4% and patient has no individual risk factors for drug resistance), EMB or SM may not be necessary and PZA may be discontinued after 2 mos.
5	Pulmonary and extrapulmonary TB in adults and children when PZA is contraindicated	9 mos	INH RIF EMB or SM**	Daily for 8 wks	INH RIF	Daily or two times wkly+ for 24 wks§	•EMB or SM should be continued until susceptibility to INH and RIF is demonstrated. •In areas where primary INH resistance is <4%, EMB or SM may not be necessary for patients with no individual risk factors for drug resistance.

* EMB = ethambutol; INH = isoniazid; PZA = pyrazinamide; RIF = rifampin; SM = streptomycin.
+ All regimens administered intermittently should be directly observed.
§ For infants and children with miliary TB, bone and joint TB, or TB meningitis, treatment should last at least 12 months. For adults with these forms of extrapulmonary TB, response to therapy should be monitored closely. If response is slow or suboptimal, treatment may be prolonged on a case-by-case basis.
¶ Some evidence suggests that SM may be discontinued after 4 months if the isolate is susceptible to all drugs.
** Avoid treating pregnant women with SM because of the risk for ototoxicity to the fetus.
Note: For all patients, if drug-susceptibility results show resistance to any of the first-line drugs or if the patient remains symptomatic or smear- or culture-positive after 3 months, consult a TB medical expert.
Source: Centers for Disease Control and Prevention (1994). Guidelines for preventing the transmission of *Mycobacterium tuberculosis* in health-care facilities, 1994. *Morbidity and Mortality Weekly Report*, 43(RR-13), p. 67.

TABLE 5.5 Dosage Recommendation for the Initial Treatment of TB Among Children[a] and Adults

	Dosage					
	Daily		2 times/week		3 times/week	
Drugs	Children	Adults	Children	Adults	Children	Adults
Isoniazid	10–20 mg/kg Max.300 mg	5 mg/kg Max. 300mg	20–40 mg/kg Max. 900mg	15 mg/kg Max 900mg	20–40 mg/kg Max. 900mg	15 mg/kg Max. 900mg
Rifampin	10 –20 mg/kg Max. 600mg	10 mg/kg Max. 600mg	10–20 mg/kg Max. 600mg	10 mg/kg Max. 600mg	10–20 mg/kg Max. 600mg	10mg/kg Max. 600mg
Pyrazin- amide	15–30 mg/kg Max.2gm	15–30 mg/kg Max.2gm	50–70 mg/kg Max.4gm	50–70 mg/kg Max.4gm	50–70 mg/kg Max 3gm	50–70 mg/kg Max.3gm
Ethambutol[b]	15–25 mg/kg Max. 2.5gm	5–25 mg/kg Max. 2.5gm	50 mg/kg Max. 2.5gm	50 gm/kg Max. 2.5gm	25–30 mg/kg Max. 2.5gm	25–30 mg/kg Max. 2.5gm
Strepto- mycin	20–30 mg/kg Max.1gm	15 mg/kg Max.1gm	25–30 mg/kg Max.1.5gm	25–30 mg/kg Max.1.5gm	25–30 mg.kg Max.1gm	25–30 mg/kg Max.1gm

[a]Children $\leq$12 years of age.
[b]Ethambutol is generally not recommended for children whose visual acuity cannot be monitored (under 6 years of age.) However, ethambutol should be considered for all children with organisms resistant to other drugs, when susceptibility to ethambutol has been demonstrated, or susceptibility is likely.

Source: Centers for Disease Control (1993). Initial therapy for tuberculosis in the era of multi–drug resistance. Recommendations of the Advisory Council for the Elimination of Tuberculosis, *Morbidity and Mortality Weekly Report, 42 (RR-7)*, p.3

culosis. These should be done quickly and accurately. To be most useful, results should be obtained within 3 to 4 weeks (Centers for Disease Control and Prevention, 1993; Mahmoudi & Iseman,

1993). These results should be reported promptly to the health department and to the health care provider.

- For initial treatment of TB, four drugs should be used. Isoniazid, rifampin, and pyrazinamide, with either ethambutol or streptomycin should be given during the first 2 months of therapy. Medications should be continued for at least 6 months and at least 3 months after sputum culture conversion to negative.
- The initial regimen should be altered on the basis of the results of drug-susceptibility testing.
- There are special circumstances that alter these recommendations. For example, low community rates (below 4%) of INH resistance may mean that fewer than four drugs can be used in the initial regimen. Places that have outbreaks of MDR-TB may need to begin with a 5-or 6-drug regimen.
- The regimen of patients with MDR-TB should be decided in consultation with physicians experienced in such treatment. If the patient is symptomatic or the culture or smear is positive after 3 months of therapy, consultation with a physician expert in MDR-TB is desirable (Centers for Disease Control and Prevention, 1993, 1994).

MDR-TB treatment is discussed later in this chapter. Treatment regimen options recommended by the CDC, using the drugs discussed earlier in this chapter, are given in Table 5.4. Recommended doses of drugs for adults and children for daily, twice-a-week, and 3-times-a-week regimens are given in Table 5.5. For patients on intermittent therapy, it is particularly important that no doses are missed.

The Tuberculosis Committee of the Infectious Diseases Society of America has initial treatment recommendations that are different from those of CDC. The group recommends a standard triple-drug regimen for persons who

1. were born in the United States;
2. live in communities that do not have a high prevalence of MDR-TB; and
3. have no known risk factors for drug-resistant TB.

The Committee states that the initial regimen may be reduced to two drugs if warranted by drug susceptibility test reports. For persons who have a slight to moderate risk of having drug-resistant TB, it recommends a four-drug regimen that includes isoniazid, rifampin, pyrazinamide, and ethambutol (Wolinsky, 1993).

Special Considerations

HIV-Infection and Immunosuppression. For patients with HIV-infection or who are otherwise immunosuppressed, the CDC currently recommends that treatment be administered for at least a total of 9 months and for at least 6 months after the sputum cultures are negative. There do not appear to be any reasons to suggest any restriction on the use of twice or 3-times-a-week administration. If drug-susceptibility results are not available, the CDC recommends continuing EMB or streptomycin for the complete therapeutic course (Centers for Disease Control and Prevention, 1993).

Extrapulmonary TB. In general, extrapulmonary TB is managed in the same way as pulmonary TB (Brausch et al., 1993) in terms of the anti-TB drug selected and dosage. Some experts believe that for those with disseminated TB, tuberculous lymphadenitis, miliary TB, or TB of the bones or joints therapy should be extended to 9 months, and that additional therapy (surgery or corticosteroids) may be useful (Centers for Disease Control and Prevention, 1993).

Pregnancy and Breast-feeding. Treatment for TB in pregnant women is important; however, it is important to choose drugs that are not harmful to the fetus. Streptomycin has been shown to have harmful fetal effects (ototoxicity), and there are inadequate data on the teratogenicity of pyrazinamide. Therefore, unless essential, PZA should not be used. The preferred initial regimen for pregnant women is isoniazid, rifampin, and ethambutol for a minimum of 9 months (Centers for Disease Control and Prevention, 1993). For women who are breast-feeding, anti-TB therapy is still recommended. It is estimated that only about 20% or less of the dose is received by the breast-feeding child. Mothers can be advised to take their medication immediately after breast-feeding and substitute a bottle at the next feeding. Breast-feeding infants do not receive protection from TB through their mother's breast milk. If they require their own treatment, then they must be carefully observed for toxicity signs and symptoms (Brausch et al., 1993).

Children. Children are treated with the same basic drug regimens (with appropriate dosage adjustments) as adults, with one exception. Because EMB can have undesirable effects on vision, and it is difficult to monitor vision in those under 6 years of age, streptomycin is often substituted. In children, sputum specimens are less likely to be useful than in adults, and so often, the results of culture and drug susceptibility test of the adult source are used to choose drugs for treatment. In some types of

TABLE 5.6 Monitoring Drug Therapy in TB

A. Baseline Evaluation/Monitoring
  1. Examination and Interview
    a. Clinical Signs and Symptoms
       Cough, productive or nonproductive
       Sputum characteristics, i.e., hemoptysis
       Fever, sweats
       Fatigue, malaise
       Anorexia
       Local signs and symptoms if extrapulmonary TB
       Others
    b. Weight
    c. Vision (acuity and red-green color perception) and hearing testing if planning
       to use drugs such as EMB or SM
    d. Presence of other conditions or medication use influencing TB therapy, i.e.,
       malnutrition, pregnancy, use of birth control pills; other
    e. Assessment for potential nonadherence
  2. Patient and Family Teaching
    a. Tuberculosis
    b. Infectivity and preventing spread—cough and handwashing techniques
    c. Drug regimen information (i.e., to expect body fluid discoloration in rifampin;
       to report any nausea, vomiting, or symptoms of INH toxicity, and what to do;
       and assessment for potential nonadherence; give at level that can be understood
       and that is culturally appropriate
  3. Laboratory
    a. Sputum culture for presence of mycobacteria
    b. Chest radiographs
    c. Blood test for liver and for renal function, such as hepatic enzymes, bilirubin,
       creatinine
    d. Complete blood count and platelets
    e. Uric acid if beginning PZA
B. Monthly Evaluation/Monitoring
  1. Evaluate clinical signs and symptoms:
    a. of disease
    b. for drug side effects or toxicity depending on drug regimen but usually including
       nausea, vomiting, jaundice, abdominal pain, fever, dark urine, numbness or
       tingling, and so on.
  2. Monitor weight
  3. Laboratory and other testing
    a. Sputum cultures for mycobacteria
    b. Blood tests to evaluate any signs or symptoms of potential drug toxicity
    c. Vision tests, auditory testing, depending on drug regimen
  4. Assess problems and answer questions
    a. Check for adherence
  5. Additional teaching as necessary

extrapulmonary TB in children (e.g., bone, joint, meningitis, disseminated), a minimum of 1 year of therapy may be used. It is important that treatment for infants and young children be thorough and immediate because of the greater risk of dissemination (American Thoracic Society, 1994; Centers for Disease Control, 1993). Dosages for children are shown in Table 5.5.

Monitoring Drug Therapy

Monitoring of patients receiving drug therapy for TB should include both clinical assessment and laboratory testing. At the beginning of therapy, baseline information should be collected or reviewed since some will have been part of the diagnostic work-up. The assessments and time period for them will vary somewhat depending upon the drug regimen selected; patient factors; access to and availability of health care and other parameters. These are summarized in Table 5.6 and are discussed also in Chapter 6. All information given to the patient and family should be culturally sensitive and competent and at a level that can be understood. Every attempt should be made to determine what potential treatment obstacles may exist for an individual and to tailor the drug regimen to an optimal plan as much as possible because nonadherence is the major reason for TB treatment failure. For patients who cannot or will not follow the treatment regimen, directly observed therapy in which a trained person actually watches the patient take medication, may be necessary as discussed in Chapters 7 and 10. A first level of drug administration that is least restrictive is the voluntary taking of medication. This is followed by potentially more restrictive techniques and settings from directly observed therapy in the home or clinic to voluntary hospitalization in a special TB unit to the most restrictive approach of compulsory hospitalization in a secure TB treatment unit (Nardell, 1993). Adherence is discussed in Chapter 7, and long-term treatment units are discussed in Chapter 13.

An important aspect to follow is the sputum culture for those patients who had positive cultures before treatment. It is generally considered that infectiousness to others decreases as the number of tubercle bacilli in the sputum decrease, and that when sputum cultures become negative, the patient is probably no longer infectious to others. Decreasing acid-fast bacilli in the sputum with eventual negativity is an indicator of successful treatment, as is the improvement in symptoms. The time period for this to occur can range from 2 weeks to 3 months, but the vast majority (90-95%) of patients become culture negative by 3 months (Barnes & Barrows, 1993; Van Scoy & Wilkowske, 1992). Patients whose sputum has not converted to negative after 5 to 6 months of therapy have been called "treatment failures" (American Thoracic Society, 1994). Chest radiographs show improvement more slowly; therefore they can be useful in monitoring progress after several months and at the conclusion of therapy (Barnes et al., 1993) Patients who continue to 1) be symptomatic or 2) have continued positive sputum cultures may have drug-resistant organisms and/or be nonadherent to their therapy. In any case, the cause must be determined so that adequate therapy can be given. Individuals with drug-susceptible TB on adequate medication with clinical resolution of symptoms and bacteriologic response to therapy are probably no longer infectious; however, there is no single universal period of time on chemotherapy that means that infectiousness ends (Centers for Disease Control and Prevention, 1994; Noble, 1981).

Relapses and Retreatment

The standard drug therapy regimen as described earlier in this chapter will be successful in the vast majority of patients with drug-susceptible TB. If relapses occur, they will generally be seen in the first year after treatment. It will be necessary to culture the sputum and do drug-susceptibility studies for optimal retreatment (O'Brien, 1993). If drug-resistant TB is found, consultation with a physician who is expert in this area is needed.

Errors in treatment can result in the development of multidrug-resistant TB and may be the responsibility of the patient, the provider, or both. Most result from inadequate treatment or nonadherence to medications. Some of these errors include

- inappropriate choice of drugs or single drug choice;
- adding a single drug to failing regimen;
- adding a single new drug after one month on regimen;
- inappropriate or irregular administration of medications;
- failure to recognize drug resistance;
- premature discontinuation of medication by patient or health care provider;
- other nonadherence to therapy (e.g., taking only one of multiple medications, decreasing dosage);
- failure of provider to suspect or recognize nonadherence to therapy;
- nonprovision of directly observed therapy in cases where nonadherence is suspected; and
- malabsorption of medication due to bowel disease or other medications (this is not uncommon in patients with HIV-disease)(Mahmoudi et al., 1993).

Other reasons for development of drug-resistant TB include host factors favorable for multiplication of resistant *M. tuberculosis*; the TB bacilli population; other host factors; pharmaceutical and pharmacological factors such as bioavailability, dispensing, or storage problems; and administrative factors such as substandard purchasing (Gangadharam, 1993).

TREATMENT OF MULTIDRUG-RESISTANT TUBERCULOSIS (MDR-TB)

MDR-TB can be defined as " . . . a case of tuberculosis caused by a strain of *Mycobacterium tuberculosis* resistant to two or more antituberculosis drugs" (Riley, 1993, p. S442), although different definitions may be found. Drug-resistant TB is a case of TB that is resistant to one anti-TB drug, most commonly isoniazid or rifampin. As discussed in Chapter 3, there is greater prevalence of MDR-TB in the United States today than previously. Appropriate chemotherapy is aimed at protecting against the emergence of drug resistant organisms.

Drug resistance can be primary (initial) or acquired (secondary) (American Thoracic Society, 1994). Primary drug resistance results from original infection with drug-resistant organisms; whereas in acquired drug resistance, strains that naturally mutate and become resistant overgrow those that are susceptible and eventually predominate. Spontaneous mutation is responsible for *Mycobacterium tuberculosis* becoming drug resistant to an anti-TB drug, and the proportion of this naturally-occurring process has been established for some of the major anti-TB drugs: isoniazid, 1 in 10^6, rifampin, 1 in 10^8, ethambutol, 1 in 10^4, and streptomycin, 1 in 10^6. The probability of resistance to two drugs occurring in the same organism spontaneously is the product of probabilities. For example, the probability of both streptomycin and rifampin resistance occurring in the same organism is 1 in 10^{14} (Centers for Disease Control and Prevention, 1993). A person with a cavitary lung lesion might harbor somewhere between 1 in 10^9 to 1 in 10^{14}, thus even in advanced disease it is not likely that *M. tuberculosis* will become resistant to two drugs if the patient is appropriately treated (Centers for Disease Control and Prevention, 1993; Riley, 1993a).

Patients who are resistant to only one antituberculous drug such as isoniazid can be successfully treated by using multiple combinations of drugs to which their organism is susceptible. It is important never to add just one drug to a failing regimen; at least two new drugs to which the organism is sensitive should be added (Riley, 1993). For example, in one study patients who were infected with organisms resistant to either isoniazid or streptomycin had treatment success rates of 94% to 96% when treated with multiple drugs over a 6-month period (Hong Kong

Chest Service/British Medical Research Council, 1987). However, reporting on a series of 171 patients with multidrug-resistant organisms at National Jewish Center, the overall favorable response rate to treatment was 56%. Of the 44% with treatment failure, 46% died from TB (Goble et al., 1993).

The implications of the inability to cure a case of multidrug-resistant TB are profound. The patient becomes a pariah of the community. Public health departments become "watchdogs," making sure the patient isn't exposing others. Directly observed therapy (DOT), if performed with initial drug-susceptible cases of TB can prevent the most common cause of drug resistant disease—nonadherence to therapy—but is not always practical or cost effective, although the benefits may outweigh these considerations. If a patient does have TB due to multidrug-resistant organisms, he may well be placed on a "last chance" regimen for cure. It is *absolutely essential* that therapy be directly observed in these cases, particularly with more toxic, long-term therapy.

Embarking upon the treatment of a case of drug-resistant TB, however, is fraught with difficulty. It is better to prevent MDR-TB than to treat it; however, that is not always possible. Important steps in beginning treatment include a detailed history of prior chemotherapy for TB and careful drug susceptibility testing on the organism (Iseman, 1993). In many cases, the course of treatment is the last chance for the patient to achieve cure and therefore must be properly initiated and managed.

For re-treatment of MDR-TB, it has been recommended that at least four, and as many as seven, drugs should be used. The number and choice depends upon disease characteristics and the drug susceptibility of the infecting organism (Iseman, 1993). In choosing a regimen, some important points are to try to: 1)include at least 3 drugs that have proven in vitro susceptibility; 2) use drugs with in vitro susceptibility that have not been used before in that patient (prior use may partially compromise susceptibility); and 3) use a regimen that the patient can tolerate. For example, health care providers should try not to use three drugs that all have severe gastrointestinal side effects (Iseman et al., 1989) because patient adherence to therapy may be compromised.

Often re-treatment for MDR-TB is best initiated within the hospital although, at first consideration, it may seem costly, in the long run, it may increase ultimate cure rates and be cost effective. Hospitalization allows incremental increases in drug dosing and timing of administration to achieve the desired peak serum concentrations with the minimum of side effects. It is also important to determine whether nonadherence was a component in prior treatment failure. If previous therapy was directly observed, then there may be other factors that led to treatment failure such as malabsorption of medications, and this can be detected during this time (Iseman, 1993). Malabsorption is common in patients with HIV disease and other conditions and can result in treatment failure (Berning, Huitt, Iseman, & Peloquin, 1992). During initial retreatment, careful monitoring of sputum specimens for semiquantitative smear and weekly culture is important. The first response indicator is improvement in bacteriologic tests of sputum because chest radiograph changes may take longer to see. Symptom improvement is another important indicator, and nurses can note and document weight gain, decreased fever, and decreased cough and sputum production (Iseman, 1993).

It is difficult to project the optimal length of time for re-treatment of MDR-TB. This depends on many factors, including the drug regimen selected and the patient response. In one center, the National Jewish Center for Immunology and Respiratory Medicine, injectable drugs may be given for 4 to 6 months, and oral medications may be given for 24 months after the sputum culture becomes negative (Iseman, 1993).

SURGICAL TREATMENT

Surgery can be an important adjunctive treatment in MDR-TB and in skeletal TB (Barnes et al., 1993; Goldsmith, 1992). Candidates for surgery in pulmonary MDR-TB include those 1) in whom several series of medical therapy have failed; 2) with persistently positive sputum samples for TB; and 3) who have extensive lung tissue destruction (Goldsmith, 1992). Before surgery, patients are on drug therapy (usually for 3 months) to reduce the mycobacterial load. It is important to have a surgeon who is experienced in this type of surgery (Goldsmith, 1992). These patients often have distorted anatomy and extensive scarring and calcification. After surgery, it is assumed that antituberculous medications will have a greater chance of coping with the fewer organisms that remain in more normal lung tissue. Postsurgical medication is usually continued for at least 2 years in MDR-TB (Goldsmith, 1992). In those with skeletal TB, surgical debridement allows anti-TB drugs to penetrate (Barnes et at., 1993).

VACCINATION

Bacille Calmette-Guérin (BCG) vaccination has enjoyed greater popularity outside the United States, although it has been used in this country, sometimes for vaccination of health-care workers. BCG consists of an attenuated strain of *M. bovis*. Successful vaccination results in a conversion to a positive tuberculin skin test, which limits the usefulness of skin testing in areas of low TB prevalence such as the United States (Dunlap & Briles, 1993). The skin test reaction to PPD resulting from BCG vaccination cannot be distinguished from a reaction resulting from infection with *M. tuberculosis* (Centers for Disease Control and Prevention, 1994). BCG vaccination is practiced elsewhere in the world. The World Health Organization has recommended the use of BCG at or shortly after birth for HIV-infected children and are asymptomatic, who are living where the risk of TB is high and where the risk of TB outweights potential complications from BCG administration; however, there is some debate about this recommendation. It is generally agreed that any child or adult who is HIV-infected and symptomatic should not receive BCG. BCG vaccination is not recommended for the general population in the United States because in communities where the risk of TB infection is low, the risks may outweigh the benefits (Pitchenik & Fertel, 1992; Quinn, 1989; ten Dam, 1993). In the United States, BCG has been recommended for infants and children who have had nonreactive skin tests under certain circumstances (Centers for Disease Control, 1988). Reconsideration of recommendations for BCG vaccine use has been prompted by the MDR-TB outbreaks (Colditz, et al. 1994) Adverse reactions to BCG have included local reactions, lymphadenitis, and rarely, osteomyelitis, erythema nodosum, disseminated BCG-itis, and others but are relatively uncommon (ten Dam, 1993).

SUMMARY

Drug therapy is the cornerstone of treatment in TB. For those with tuberculous infection, preventive drug therapy may be indicated. For drug-susceptible TB, in persons without HIV infection a combination of isoniazid, rifampin, pyrazidaminde, and ethambutol or streptomycin can be administered in a variety of schedules for at least 6 months, and the chance for successful treatment is excellent. A major reason for the development of MDR-TB is treatment failure due to inadequate or inappropriate treatment or nonadherence. No drug treatment can be successful if the drug does "not enter the patient's body" (American Thoracic Society, 1994, p. 1361) or is not taken according to the appropriate plan. Ways to ensure completion of the regimen, such as directly observed therapy may be necessary. The treatment of MDR-TB can be complicated and fraught with difficulty but necessary. Surgical resection can be used in conjunction with medication.

REFERENCES

American Thoracic Society (1990). Diagnostic standards and classification of tuberculosis. *American Review of Respiratory Disease, 142,* 725–735.

American Thoracic Society (1992). Control of tuberculosis in the United States.*American Review of Respiratory Disease 146,* 1623–1633.

American Thoracic Society. (1994). Treatment of tuberculosis and tuberculosis infection in adults and children. *American Journal of Respiratory and Critical Care Medicine, 149,* 1359–1374

Ballow, C. H., Chapman, S. W., & Martin, D. H. (1993). The new macrolides: Beyond erythromycin. *Patient Care, 27(20),* 125–136.

Barnes, P. F. & Barrows, S. A. (1993).Tuberculosis in the 1990s. *Annals of Internal Medicine, 119,* 400–410.

Barnes, P. F., Le, H. Q., & Davidson, P. T. (1993). Tuberculosis in patients with HIV infection. *Medical Clinics of North America, 77(6),* 1369–1390.

Berning, S.E., Huitt, G.A., Iseman, M.D., & Peloquin, C.A. (1992). Malabsorption of antituberculosis medications by a patient with AIDS. *New England Journal of Medicine, 327,*1817–1818.

Brausch, L. M., & Bass, J. B. Jr. (1993). The treatment of tuberculosis. *Medical Clinics of North America, 77(6),* 1277–1288.

Center for Disease Control. (1988). Use of BCG vaccines in the control of tuberculosis: A joint statement by the ACIP and the Advisory Committee for Elimination of Tuberculosis. *Morbidity and Mortality Weekly Report, 37,* 663–675.

Center for Disease Control and Prevention (1992). Management of persons exposed to multidrug-resistant tuberculosis. *Morbidity and Mortality Weekly Report, 41(No. RR-11),* 61–71.

Centers for Disease Control and Prevention (1993). Initial therapy for tuberculosis in the era of multidrug resistance. *Morbidity and Mortality Weekly Report, 42 (No.RR-7),* 1–8.

Centers for Disease Control. (1994). Guidelines for preventing the transmission of *Mycobacterium tuberculosis* in health-care facilities, 1994. *Morbidity and Mortality Weekly Report, 43* (RR-13), 1–133.

Colditz, G. A., Brewer, T. F., Berkey, C. S., Wilson, M. E., Burdick, E., Fineberg, H. V., & Mosteller, F. (1994). Efficacy of BCG vaccine in the prevention of tuberculosis: Meta-analysis of the published literature. *Journal of the American Medical Association, 271,* 598–702.

DiFerdinando, G. T. Jr., Glassroth, J., Hecht, F. M., & Stover, D. E. (1993). TB and HIV: A deadly synergy. *Patient Care, 27(14),* 92–114.

Ebert, S. C.(1989). Tuberculosis. In DiPiro, J. T., Talbert, R. L., Hayes, P. E., Yee, G. C. & Posey, L.M.(Eds.).*Pharmacotherapy: A pathophysiologic approach.* (pp 153–1165). New York, Elsevier.

Ellner, J. J., Hinman, A. R., Dooley, S. W., Fischl, M. A., Sepkowitz, K.

A., Goldberger, M. J., Shinnick, T. M., Iseman, M. D., & Jacobs, W. R., Jr. (1993). Tuberculosis symposium: Emerging problems and promise. *Journal of Infectious Diseases, 168,* 537–531.

Gangadharam, P. R. J. (1993). Drug resistance in tuberculosis. *Lung Biology in Health and Disease, 66,* 293–328.

Geiter, L. J. (1993). Preventive therapy for tuberculosis. *Lung Biology in Health and Disease, 66,* 241–250.

Goble, M., Iseman, M.D., Madsen, L.A., Waite, D., Ackerson, L., Horsburgh, R.C. (1993). Treatment of 171 patients with pulmonary tuberculosis resistant to isoniazid and rifampin. *New England Journal of Medicine, 328,* 527–532.

Goldsmith, M. F. (1992). Surgeons say cutting out some TB and MOTT may be the answer in multidrug-resistant infections. *Journal of the American Medical Association, 268,* 3178–3179.

Hong Kong Chest Service/British Medical Research Council (1987). Five-year follow-up of a controlled trial of five 6-month regimens of chemotherapy for pulmonary tuberculosis. *American Review of Respiratory Disease, 136,* 1339–1342.

Iseman, M. D. (1993). Treatment of multidrug-resistant tuberculosis. *New England Journal of Medicine, 329,* 784–791.

Iseman, M.D.,& Madsen, L.A. (1989). Drug resistant tuberculosis. *Clinics in Chest Medicine. 10 (3),*341–353.

Madsen, L.A., Berning, S.E. (1993). Tolerance to the fluoroquinolone antibiotics in the treatment of mycobacterial disease. Poster presented at the American Thoracic Society Meeting, San Francisco, CA, May, 1993.

Mahmoudi, A. & Iseman, M. D. (1993). Pitfalls in the care of patients with tuberculosis. *Journal of the American Medical Association, 270,* 65–68.

Mandell, G. L., Douglas, R. G. Jr., & Bennett, J. (Eds) (1990). *Principles and Practice of Infectious Diseases.* (3rd ed.). New York: Churchill Livingstone.

Mandell, G. L., & Sande, M. A. (1990). Antimicrobial agents. Drugs used in the chemotherapy of tuberculosis and leprosy. In Gilman, A. G., Rall, T. W., Nies, A. S. & Taylor, P. (Eds.). *Goodman and Gilman's The pharmacological basis of therapeutics.* (8th ed., pp. 1146–1164). New York: Pergamon Press.

Miller, B. (1993). Preventive therapy for tuberculosis. *Medical Clinics of North America, 77(6),* 1263–1275.

Nardell, E. A. (1993). Beyond four drugs. *American Review of Respiratory Disease, 148,* 2–5.

Noble, R.C. (1981). Infectiousness of pulmonary tuberculosis after starting chemotherapy. *American Journal of Infection Control, 9,* 6–10.

O'Brien, R. J. (1993). The treatment of tuberculosis. *Lung Biology in Health and Disease, 66,* 207–240.

Peloquin, C. A. (1993). Pharmacology of the antimycobacterial drugs. *Medical Clinics of North America, 77(6),* 1253–1262.

Peloquin, C. A. & Berning, S. E. (1994). Infection caused by *Mycobacterium tuberculosis. The Annals of Pharmacotherapy, 28,* 72–84.

Perez-Stable, E. J., & Hopewell, P. C. (1989). Current tuberculosis treatment regimens. *Clinics in Chest Medicine, 10(3)*, 323–339.

Physicians' Desk Reference. (1994). 48th edition. Montvale, New Jersey: Medical Economics Data.

Riley, L. W. (1993). Drug-resistant tuberculosis. *Clinical Infectious Diseases, 17(Suppl 2)*, S442–S446.

Snider, D. E., & Caras, G. J. (1992). Isoniazid-associated hepatitis deaths: A review of the available information. *American Review of Respiratory Disease, 145*, 484–497.

ten Dam, H. G. (1993). BCG vaccination. *Lung Biology in Health and Disease, 66*, 251–273.

Van Scoy, R. E., & Wilkowske, C. J. (1992). Antituberculous agents. *Mayo Clinic Proceedings, 67*, 179–187.

Wolinsky, E. (1993). Statement of the tuberculosis committee of the Infectious Diseases Society of America. *Clinical Infectious Diseases, 16*, 627–628.

6

NURSING MANAGEMENT OF TUBERCULOSIS

Helena Sibilano

Nurses have always played key roles in the care for persons with tuberculosis (TB). Nurses today carry out numerous TB-related activities: case-finding, surveillance, case management, acute care management, primary care, prevention activities (including contact tracing), patient, family, and community education, and research (Black & Matassarin-Jacobs, 1993; Daugherty, Hutton, & Simone, 1993). These activities are implemented in a wide variety of settings, including hospitals, nursing homes, outpatient and specialty clinics, and other health care institutions; occupational settings; public health agencies; and community settings. Wherever TB is an actual or potential health problem, nurses will be found on the front line. This chapter provides an overview of nursing management of the person with TB and related supplemental materials.

ACUTE CARE MANAGEMENT

Although most of the care of patients with TB occurs in the community (see Chapter 10), patients may also be in the acute care setting. The

99

professional nurse must maintain a "high index of suspicion" to identify a potentially infectious TB patient. The "known" TB patient is placed on TB isolation (described later in chapter 9) and antituberculosis medications, thus reducing the possibility of airborne transmission of TB to others; however, the patient with other admitting diagnoses such as pneumonia, weight loss, cancer of the lung, or diabetes could also have active, infectious TB. Such patients can be hospitalized for long periods before the accurate diagnosis of TB is finally made. In some cases, TB is revealed only by autopsy. Meanwhile, health care personnel, roommates, and visitors have already been exposed to contaminated air. Now, more than ever, with multidrug resistant TB (MDR-TB), prompt early diagnosis is essential to prevent spread of TB.

The Tuberculosis Index of Suspicion Tool (TIST)

The tuberculosis index of suspicion tool (TIST) was developed and has been used clinically by the author as a nursing assessment tool (see Figure 6.1). This tool is designed to assist the professional nurse, working in any setting, in identifying infectious, active TB patients. The nurse completes the TIST immediately after admission of a new patient into any setting, such as a nursing home, hospital, or shelter.

First, frequent signs and symptoms associated with active TB are listed. The nurse completes this column, noting their presence or absence in the patient. Whenever the symptom of cough is checked, a diagnostic investigation for TB is indicated. The nurse then categorizes the patient according to membership in the high-risk groups. The nurse should strive to display sensitivity, a nonjudgmental attitude and strict confidence in gathering information, particularly from members of high-risk groups. The nurse then analyzes the information gathered by the number of checks in the "yes" column, the outcome being that the patient is categorized as having a low or high index of suspicion for TB infection or disease (see chapters 3,4, and 5).

TB Isolation

Once the nurse determines that the patient has a high index of suspicion for TB, TB isolation should be initiated during the diagnostic testing period to protect staff and others (see Chapter 9 and Centers for Disease Control and Prevention, 1994). The nurse monitors negative pressure as part of the isolation components:

- A private room with negative air pressure preventing the air in the room from going back out into the hospital corridor.

SYMPTOM

	Yes	No
Cough: Non-productive	□	□
Cough: Productive	□	□
Night Sweats	□	□
Weight Loss	□	□
Anorexia	□	□
Fatigue	□	□
Weakness	□	□
Fever/Chills	□	□
Hemoptysis	□	□

MEMBER OF HIGH RISK GROUP

	Yes	No
HIV Positive/AIDS	□	□
History of Tuberculosis	□	□
History of Positive PPD Skin Test	□	□
Adolescent < 15 years	□	□
Elderly > 65 years	□	□
Poverty/Homeless	□	□

High Risk Group cont.

	Yes	No
Community Living:		
Prison, Nursing Home, Shelter	□	□
Alcohol/Drug Abuse	□	□
Recent Exposure to "active"		
TB case	□	□
Recent immigration:		
Asia, Africa, South America	□	□
Pneumonia	□	□
Health Care Worker,		
Prison Security Guard	□	□
Chronic illness:		
• Silicosis	□	□
• diabetes mellitus	□	□
• chronic immunosuppressive therapy	□	□
• hematologic diseases (leukemia)	□	□
• end-stage renal disease	□	□
• intestinal bypass	□	□
• post-gastrectomy	□	□
• chronic malabsorption syndrome	□	□
• CA of mouth and GI tract	□	□
• 10% or below ideal body weight	□	□

Diagnostic Workup:

• Screen "suspicious" patient with cough of undetermined origin:

• PPD skin test induration: _____ mm.

• Anergy battery: Placement of 3 common environmental antigens in opposite arm of PPD skin test to verify that patients immune system is functioning adequately: especially indicated with HIV/AIDS and elderly populations.

• Mumps: _____ mm. Candida: _____ mm. Other: _____ mm.

• Sputum Smear: (test results available within 24 hours; send minimum of three)
  Positive AFB _____ Negative AFB _____

• Sputum Culture/Sensitivity Study: (test results available in 4 to 8 weeks)
  Positive _____ Organism _____

• TB isolation: Yes □   No □

• Chest X-ray: Normal _____ Abnormal _____ Cavitary _____

• Instructed patient on cough/sneeze protection technique:
  Cooperative _____ Uncooperative _____

FIGURE 6.1 Tuberculosis Index of Suspicion Nursing Assessment Tool

- A gauge outside room indicating negative pressure within the room; engineering department responsible for periodic checks on adequate functioning of system.
- Six to eight complete air exchanges per hour within the room, as verified by the engineering department.
- The air within the room is exhausted directly to the outside and away from a re-entry vent to prevent recirculation of droplet nuclei.
- Doors and windows kept closed at all times to maintain negative pressure within the room.
- Patient uses proper sneeze/cough technique to reduce airborne contamination (discussed in the next section).

All health care personnel and visitors entering the room should use the recommended respiratory protective device; the patient wears a well-fitted mask whenever leaving the room for any special tests or procedures; otherwise, patients should remain in their rooms at all times (Centers for Disease Control and Prevention, 1994). TB isolation precautions must be officially discontinued before the patient is allowed to visit throughout the hospital freely. Criteria for the discontinuation of TB isolation may vary among institutions and practitioners. This cannot be a blanket period of time but must include an evaluation of the patient's response to the anti-TB medications; clinical improvement including a reduction in coughing and absence of fever; and a progressive reduction in the number of acid-fast bacilli (AFB) in the sputum smear (three negative sputums collected on 3 consecutive days (Centers for Disease Control and Prevention, 1994). However, the decision to discontinue TB isolation should be individually determined. The patient should then be transferred to a private room until discharge. The TB patient should never be transferred to a room with a patient who has HIV-infection or another type of immunosuppression.

Cough/Sneeze Protection Technique

The actively coughing and expectorating patient is treated as infectious and should be categorized as having a high index of suspicion for TB. Coughing and sneezing generate large numbers of respiratory droplets, many of which evaporate into droplet nuclei and become vehicles for airborne TB transmission. Because droplet nuclei are small (1–5 microns), air currents can keep them airborne for hours.

The nurse should demonstrate the cough/sneeze protection technique to the patient and family. The patient covers both nose and mouth with

TABLE 6.1 Nursing Care Plan for Persons with Suspected or Confirmed Tuberculosis*

I. Subjective-Assessment
   A. History of presenting signs and symptoms (refer to TB Index of Suspicion Tool) (TIST)
   B. History of previous tuberculosis treatment
      —length of time
      —medication taken
      —treatment outcome
   C. History of exposure to person with tuberculosis
      —when
      —relationship
      —did person have multidrug-resistant TB
   D. Other coexisting conditions, e.g., diabetes mellitus, chronic bronchitis, cancer
   E. History of smoking and alcohol and drug use
   F. Patient's close contacts
   G. Current medications

II. Objective-Assessment
   A. Review of all body systems with emphasis on respiratory assessment
   B. Vital signs
   C. Weight/height
   D. Sputum: amount, color, consistency

III. Short-term Goals
   A. Prevent transmission of tuberculosis to others
   B. Implement TB isolation
   C. Begin antituberculosis medication regimen
   D. Begin patient and family education
   E. Teach cough/sneeze protection technique
   F. Prevent complications due to disease or therapy
   G. Report to local board of health for contact tracing, testing, and follow-up

IV. Long-term Goals
   A. Cure TB by an adequate antituberculosis medication treatment plan over an adequate time period
   B. Enhance adherence and cooperation of patient and family
   C. Prevent development of multidrug-resistant tuberculosis (MDR-TB)
   D. Continue education of patient and family about tuberculosis and treatment regimen
   E. Assist patient in improving overall health by dealing with concurrent problems, e.g., alcohol/drug abuse, HIV-infection

*These are areas of emphasis for TB patients. A complete standard nursing assessment should be performed including psychological, social, and other aspects.

tissue whenever coughing or sneezing. This is the most important step in preventing the transmission of TB because this disease is mainly transmitted by airborne droplet nuclei containing *Mycobacterium tuberculo-*

sis. All health-care workers should follow this same technique and role-model proper sneeze/cough protection. The patient should be given an adequate supply of tissues at the bedside and should carry tissues whenever leaving the room. Soiled tissue should be discarded in a container after which hands are thoroughly washed.

Nursing Care of the Acutely Ill Tuberculosis Patient

Persons who are very ill, experiencing complications, or needing complex tests for diagnosis are hospitalized. Hospitalization is usually brief, involving care continued on an ambulatory basis with a referral for community nursing. A few patients may require prolonged institutional care where directly observed therapy (DOT) can be accomplished. (see Chapters 10 and 13). Nursing diagnoses commonly seen in patients with TB are in Appendix 6A.

The nurse should individualize a plan of care according to the severity of the patient's disease and complications and other medical, psychological, and social problems and involve both the patient and family in the care process. Nursing approaches in providing care for persons with active TB are outlined in Table 6.1. In conclusion, the nurse identifies, isolates, and begins treatment of active tuberculosis patients as early as possible, thereby decreasing the risk of TB transmission to others in the environment. The patient benefits by early diagnosis and treatment, thus decreasing the risk of complications and mortality.

TESTING AND DIAGNOSIS

Tuberculin Skin Test/Anergy Battery

Nurses play important roles in screening for tuberculosis. It bears emphasizing that the most commonly used tuberculin skin test, the Mantoux (sometimes called PPD), only signifies infection with *Mycobacterium*. This test is not diagnostic of active TB (Amin, 1994, Avey, 1993; Huebner, Schein, & Bass, 1993). The Mantoux test must be correctly administered and interpreted (see Chapter 8).

Chest Radiography

Chest radiography is indicated if there is a suspicion of TB. However, tuberculosis is seldom diagnosed solely on radiographic results since other diseases can mimic tuberculosis radiographically. Radiography is discussed in Chapter 4. A cavitary lesion in patients with a high index of suspicion of TB indicates the possibility of a large population of live *M. tuberculosis*, about one billion organisms per lesion. Therefore, isolation precautions are often maintained longer in TB patients with cavitary lesions than they would otherwise be.

Sputum Collection and Examination

The nurse should collect a minimum of three sputum specimens for AFB smear and for culture and sensitivity to confirm pulmonary tuberculosis in the high index of suspicion patient. Sputum specimens are collected on 3 consecutive mornings as soon as patient awakens. The patient is instructed to cough up secretions from deep within the chest. Several deep breaths will often stimulate effective coughing. Sputum specimens are collected in a negative pressure isolation room or specially designed booths to prevent spread. No one else should be present in the room or booth. These booths should not be used for another patient until adequate time has passed so that the ventilation system has removed droplet nuclei. This time will vary according to the efficiency of the system (Centers for Disease Control and Prevention, 1994).

Sometimes a patient is unable to produce sputum. A pooled sputum specimen may then collected over a period of 12 to 24 hours (although many laboratories will not accept these specimens because of the over-growth of other organisms), or a sputum specimen is induced using aerosolized hypertonic saline. Sputum specimens are also obtained dur-ing bronchoscopy examination. At times, an early morning aspiration of gastric contents is necessary to obtain sputum. AFB smear, culture, and sensitivity examination may be ordered on the appropriate tissue or fluid (such as pleural fluid, peritoneal fluid, spinal fluid, blood, or urine) whenever extrapulmonary tuberculosis is suspected (MacGregor, 1993; Roberts & Thompson, 1994). It is important that the nurse ensure proper and prompt handling of the specimens.

The nurse monitors sputum AFB smear results, which are available within 24 hours. A negative sputum smear does not rule out tuberculosis; however, a negative sputum smear does indicate a low degree of infect-ivity to others. Conversely, a positive sputum smear with AFB indicates potential infectivity to others. Isolation precautions remain in effect until three sputum smear results are negative and other criteria are met (see chapters 5 and 9).

Because *M. tuberculosis* is slow growing, a sputum *culture* can take 6 to 8 weeks to show results. However, a positive culture for *Mycobacte-*

rium tuberculosis is considered a definitive diagnosis for tuberculosis disease. The nurse should follow up on the sputum culture results to verify tuberculosis. The drug sensitivity results from sputum cultures assist the practitioner in determining which drugs will be most effective in treating the patient. A copy of a positive culture and sensitivity report should be sent to the public health agencies according to local and state laws and agency protocols.

COMMUNITY NURSE ROLE

The TB patient is usually treated as an outpatient, unless the medical condition warrants hospitalization. Because family members and others living or working in close proximity, have already been exposed to the patient's most infectious period, all those exposed by close contact must also be considered potentially infected. The community health nurse (CHN) may begin the contact investigation, which is described in Chapter 10.

The community health nurse (CHN) makes the home environment safer through assessment of the home environment and patient and family education about the airborne transmission of the tubercle bacilli. Proper cough and sneeze protection technique is demonstrated to the patient and family members who should return the demonstration. The patient is instructed to follow this technique even when alone because airborne droplet nuclei contaminate the air for hours.

When collecting a sputum specimen, the patient should be instructed to cough into the container either outside the home in open air or in a room that can then be ventilated with fresh air. Others should not be present during or after this procedure until after the room is well ventilated. Ventilation of the home is encouraged to allow fresh air exchanges, thereby reducing the concentration of tuberculosis bacilli in the air; however, the comfort of the patient and family has to be considered.

When possible, parents should send children to relatives during the first 2 weeks that the patient is taking antituberculosis medications. During this time, visitors, especially children and those at high risk of contracting TB, should not be allowed to visit. The CHN should wear a protective respiratory device during the initial phase of the treatment program, discontinuing its use after the patient is determined to be noninfectious (see Chapters 9 and 10). One of the most effective infection control measures is strict implementation of sneeze and cough protection technique using tissues.

The CHN should educate the patient and the family members on all aspects of TB disease and treatment. A sample teaching plan is shown in

Appendix 6B. To help the patient remember and adhere to the medication regimen, one family member can be recruited to observe and document the patient taking all medications. The CHN can also arrange the time of home visits to witness the patient taking his medications (DOT) and to reinforce education on medications.

The CHN should complete an assessment that includes a review of signs and symptoms of TB and the common side effects of medications that the patient is taking (see Chapter 5). During contact with the patient, the CHN should measure and record vital signs and weight and collect sputum specimens periodically to monitor infectivity by the presence or absence of acid-fast bacilli. Periodic chest radiography is also indicated to assess improvement. The nurse should also attempt to assess adherence and try to use incentives and enablers to enhance adherence (see Chapter 9).

The patient can usually return to work based upon assessment of the following: (a) three sputum smear examinations are negative for AFB; (b) the antituberculosis medication regimen has been administered for a minimum of 2 weeks; (c) overall physical condition is improved and symptoms have decreased; (d) patient practices sneeze and cough protection technique consistently; and (e) the work environment is assessed as low risk for disease transmission (e.g., the tree trimmer who works outdoors).

NURSE SPECIALIST-MANAGED TUBERCULOSIS CLINIC

Outpatient TB clinics managed by nurses have been shown to be superior to general clinics in providing completely documented follow-up (Werhane, Snukst-Torbeck, & Schraufnagel, 1989). Some of these clinics are managed by nurses working in advanced nursing practice roles of nurse practitioner or clinical nurse specialist. The nurse case manager implements a plan of care that focuses upon the patient's adherence to the therapeutic regimen, particularly prescribed medications. The nurse can provide patient support and assistance, resolve blocks to adherence, help the patient to use all resources available to complete the medication regimen, and participate fully in the plan of care (also see Chapters 9 and 10).

The TB nurse commonly manages the care of patients receiving preventive therapy as discussed in Chapter 5 (e.g., isoniazid [INH]) and of active TB patients receiving standard antituberculosis medications. At the initial visit, the physician and nurse both evaluate the patient, who then typically begins to take medications according to a standard medication protocol. Thereafter, the patient is evaluated monthly by the same nurse specialist. Included in the monthly assessment are symptom evaluation, monitoring for drug side effects, and reinforcing teaching, for example, of cough/sneeze protective technique. A monitoring tool is given in Chapter 5.

The physician is involved in any changes in therapy as well as the decision to discontinue therapy, review chest radiographs, examine laboratory data, and evaluate of other medical problems. Missed appointments are rescheduled immediately. Active TB patients who do not adhere to the medical regimen are referred to the public health department for rapid follow-up. The strength of this program is the consistent relationship and continuity of care provided by physician-nurse team to the patient and family.

CONCLUSION

Nursing has a long and rich history of providing care for persons with TB in specialized settings, hospitals, and the community. Although effective drugs exist to treat TB, the emergence of multidrug-resistant TB and the HIV epidemic, coupled with other socioeconomic problems of contemporary society, has created new challenges for nurses in the ancient battle against TB. Today, nurses, as case managers and providers of primary care, are assuming key roles in treating persons with TB and in preventing the spread of this disease. Nurses, with their specialized knowledge base and high level of patient acceptance and trust, must participate as full partners in this nation's efforts to eliminate and prevent the suffering associated with tuberculosis.

APPENDIX 6A Nursing Diagnoses and Interventions for Patients With TB

Nursing Diagnosis	Expected Outcomes	Nursing Interventions
Potential for Transmission of Pulmonary Tuberculosis		

Supporting Data:

• Sputum smear positive for AFB organisms	• Prevention of "outbreak" of tuberculosis in an institutional setting	• Administer and supervise antituberculosis medication regimen
• Possibility of multidrug-resistant organism (confirmation takes 4 to 8 weeks)	• Decreasing infectivity through antituberculosis medications/therapy	• Initiate appropriate negative-pressure TB isolation precautions based on high index of suspicion assessment
• Presence of coughing or sneezing	• Cooperation with cough and sneeze protection technique	• Request hospital personnel entering the room wear a protective respiratory device; patient wears mask whenever leaving the hospital room
• Unable or unwilling to cover nose and mouth with tissue during coughing and sneezing	• Appropriate isolation technique implemented	• Keep confined to TB isolation room with doors and windows closed at all times to maintain negativity; others should limit time spent in the room.
• Increased concentration of infecting organism in the air occurring during suctioning, aerosolized treatment, bronchoscopy, and collection of sputum for examination		• Teach proper cough and protection technique
• Improper ventilation system in institution		• Educate all persons before entering patient's room on TB isolation precautions; post sign on door for all visitors to check with nurse before entering room
• Presence of pulmonary lesion(s) on x-ray		• Educate others, (e.g., dietary assistants) that telephone, tables, bed, clothing, dishes are not sources of TB and thus requires no special precautions or disinfecting procedure
• Delay in implementing isolation precautions		

Appendix 6A, continued

Nursing Diagnosis	Expected Outcomes	Nursing Interventions
		• Discontinue isolation precautions based upon a case-by-case physician or institutional determination which may include: 1) three negative AFB sputum smears, 2) evidence of reversal of clinical signs and symptoms of infection (decreased cough, sputum production, temperature, and increased appetite, weight, and absence of night sweats), 3) and adequate antituberculosis medications administered for a minimum of 2 weeks or more; chest radiography demonstrates improvement and absence of cavitary lesion(s).
		• Continue TB isolation precautions: 1) if multidrug-resistant organism is suspected, 2) patient's clinical condition is minimally improved, 3) cavitary lesion(s) remain on chest radiography, and 4) AFB organisms persist in sputum smear test
		• Institute precautions during all cough generating procedures such as an adequate ventilation system and wearing of personal respiratory protective device
		• Discharge patient to home or to another institution if facilities do not have isolation rooms available.

Appendix 6A, continued

Nursing Diagnosis	Expected Outcomes	Nursing Interventions

Potential for Impaired Gas Exchange

Nursing Diagnosis	Expected Outcomes	Nursing Interventions
Supporting Data: • Extensive disease of one or both lungs • Pneumonia • Pleural effusion • Fibrosis of lungs • Presence of other acute or chronic lung conditions, e.g., chronic obstructive pulmonary disease (COPD)	• Arterial Blood Gases (ABG) within normal limits (WNL) • Lungs clear • Oxygen saturation greater than 90% • Vital signs WNL • Improved chest x-ray • Decrease or absence of dyspnea • Decreased anxiety.	• Monitor ABG results daily and prn • Observe, report, and document signs and symptoms of hypoxia and/or hypercapnia — restlessness, anxiety — increased dyspnea — increased or decreased respiratory rate — increased heart rate — personality change (belligerent) — change in level of consciousness — excessive lethargy or somnolence • Monitor oxygen saturation • Administer oxygen therapy, as indicated • Measure level of dyspnea with an acceptable rating scale every shift • Auscultate lungs • Monitor vital signs q 4 hours and prn • Avoid use of sedatives and tranquilizers • Directly observed patient taking antituberculosis medications and document • Observe for signs and symptoms of infection: elevated temperature; change in sputum (color/amount) character

Appendix 6A, continued

Nursing Diagnosis	Expected Outcomes	Nursing Interventions
Ineffective Airway Clearance		

Supporting Data:

• Excessive mucous production due to infection • Weak, ineffective cough • Hemoptysis • Smoking	• Decreased sputum production • Effective coughing and ability to clear airway of secretions • No evidence of hemoptysis • Lungs clear • Smoking cessation	• Record sputum production, amount, color, consistency, odor • If coughing up blood, sedate and reassure • Place on affected side to minimize blood entering other lung • Control and suppress cough • Increase fluid intake to 2,000 cc daily within the level of cardiac reserve • Assess lung sounds every 8 hours and prn • Assess vital signs every 4 hours • Observe for obstruction of airway/respiratory distress • Teach effective coughing and airway clearance of secretions • Suction as needed • Encourage movement/ ambulation to facilitate mobilization and expectoration of secretions • Encourage smoking cessation and avoidance of environmental pollutants • Prepare for thoracotomy, if necessary, to control problem with hemoptysis.

Appendix 6A, continued

Nursing Diagnosis	Expected Outcomes	Nursing Interventions
Alteration in Nutrition; Less Than Body Requirement		
Supporting Data: • Anorexia • Weight loss • Wasting of muscle mass • Evidence of starvation • Abnormal laboratory data.	• Demonstrate 2 pound weight gain per week • Reaches ideal weight • Able to obtain food posthospitalization • Laboratory data within normal limits.	• Consult dietitian • Assess dietary habits and needs • Record amount of food intake • Record weight 3 times/ week • Assess need for frequent feedings • Educate patient and family to maintain optimum weight through suggested dietary program • Give high calorie liquid supplemental feeding • Gastric tube feedings/ intravenous hyperalimentation only if patient unable to take oral feeding • Assess food sources and abilities to prepare meals postdischarge.
Potential for Alteration of Fluid Volume		
Supporting Data: • Anorexia • Elevated temperature • Diaphoresis • Nausea/vomiting • Skin turgor	•.Electrolytes WNL • Hydrated skin and mucous membrane • Secretions thin	• Assess for signs of dehydration, such as poor skin turgor, dry skin, and mucous membrane • Control nausea/vomiting • Offer antiemetics • Provide frequent oral hygiene • Weigh three times per week • Encourage small frequent meals • Monitor intake and output • Administer IV fluids if necessary to provide fluid and electrolyte balance • If diaphoretic, keep bed linens dry.

Appendix 6A, continued

Nursing Diagnosis	Expected Outcomes	Nursing Interventions

Potential Risk for Acquiring Hospital-Transmitted Infection

Supporting Data:		
• Chronic disease • Malnutrition • Weakened immune system	• Absence of hospital-acquired infections	• Use scrupulous aseptic technique when doing procedures • Wash hands before each contact with patient • Keep patient separated from other patients and staff with infectious conditions • Monitor for evidence of acquired infection, e.g., increased temperature, increased white blood cell count.

Self-Care Deficit

Supporting Data:		
• Infectious process • Increased work of breathing • Weakness, fatigue, weight loss • Elevated temperature	• Decreased dyspnea • Demonstrates increased independence in self-care • Utilizes energy-conservation techniques.	• Provide physical conditioning program at the bedside and later in physical therapy department • Institute energy conservation techniques: tub bench, shower hose, alternating periods of rest and activity • Refer to social service for consideration of home health aide • Teach patient to pace activity and simplify workload.

Knowledge Deficit

Supporting Data:		
• Unable to explain disease process, treatment, medications • Demonstrates unhealthy lifestyle	• Demonstrates knowledge of disease and treatment • States names, dosages, and side effects of medications • Knows how to respond to an adverse drug effect • Knowledge of maintaining overall health.	• Discuss disease process with patient and family • Analyze how patient possibly got tuberculosis disease • Institute teaching plan (see Appendix 6B).

Appendix 6A, continued

Nursing Diagnosis	Expected Outcomes	Nursing Interventions
Potential for Ineffective Coping With Social Isolation		

Supporting Data:		
• Enforcement of isolation precaution for 2 weeks or longer	• Cooperation with AFB isolation order • Decreased depression • Decreased boredom	• Provide recreational activities, books, television, radio • Encourage short visits with a person properly protected with mask • Institute tuberculosis teaching plan and reinforce daily • If weather permits, allow trips outdoors.

Potential for Inability to Adhere to Long-Term Treatment Program		

Supporting Data:		
• Knowledge deficit • Denial of having disease • Alcoholism/drug addiction • Lack of motivation • Lack of transportation • Clinic inaccessibility • Financial problems • Homelessness • Unknown etiology	• Appointments kept • Prescriptions filled • Evidence of decreased disease process, e.g., negative sputum smears and improved chest x-ray • Cure of disease within allotted time frame • Absence of alcohol/drug abuse.	• Teach patients and family aspects of disease process and treatment • Reinforce "cure" of tuberculosis by adherence to treatment plan • Listen to patient identify what potential barriers interfere with completion of treatment program and problem solve • Find shelter for a homeless person; obtain alcohol/drug counseling and treatment; seek funds for transportation, medication, foods, and housing • Provide continuity of care by same physician/nurse team supervision throughout treatment program • Remind patient about clinic appointments and medication adherence via phone or mail

Appendix 6A, continued

Nursing Diagnosis	Expected Outcomes	Nursing Interventions
		• Provide interpreter and bilingual/bicultural staff to interpret treatment protocol and gain patient/family cooperation
		• Obtain current address and phone number at each visit contact family members and friends, if necessary, to get patient back into treatment
		• Notify local board of health of a patient lost to follow-up visits
		• Arrange intermittent DOT with visiting nurse, board of health personnel, family member, or other. This person observes and records the patient taking the antituberculosis medications 2 or 3 days a week.
		• Monitor adherence via — continued negative sputum smears — improvement in chest x-ray and symptoms — serum and urine levels of medication — pill counts — diary or self-report.
		• Start entire treatment course over as day "1" if patient has had a significant interruption of chemotherapy; may take two or three restarts before patient is able to complete entire treatment plan
		• Reevaluate drug susceptibility of organism and have medications adjusted.

Appendix 6A, continued

Nursing Diagnosis	Expected Outcomes	Nursing Interventions

**Alteration in Comfort Related to
Pleurisy/Pleural Effusion[1]**

Supporting Data:
- Chills
- Fever
- Cough
- Pain described as severe, sharp, and knifelike
- Pain worse on inspiration and coughing
- Reduced chest wall movement
- Presence of pleural friction rub
- Absence of breath sounds
- Dull percussion over affected area.

- Absorption of effusion as evidenced by improved chest x-ray
- Absence of signs and symptoms of respiratory distress
- Decreased pain
- Breath sounds WNL

- Auscultate lungs every 2 to 4 hours
- Administer antituberculosis medications
- Assist with thoracentesis to remove excess fluid and to improve ventilation
- Send pleural fluid to laboratory for cytology, smear, culture, and sensitivity
- Encourage deep breathing
- Position patient for optimum lung expansion
- Observe patient closely for any signs or symptoms of respiratory distress
- Institute adequate pain management program
- Observe for signs and symptoms of complications postthoracentesis (shock/hemo/pneumothorax

---

[1]Acute or chronic inflammation of the pleural space; effusion refers to liquid in the pleural space.

Appendix 6B Tuberculosis Teaching/Learning Protocol

Target Audience:
All tuberculosis patients and their families or significant others.

Objectives:
Patient and family will be able to
— State how tuberculosis is transmitted to others;
— Describe the mechanism of disease process;
— Demonstrate knowledge of medication protocol and length of time of treatment program;
— List names of medications and dosage;
— State side effects of medications;
— Describe what action to take when experiencing a drug side effect;
— Demonstrate knowledge of clinic visit date and time;
— List name and phone number of pulmonary clinical nurse specialist and physician.

Content:
— Cough/sneeze precaution technique;
— Tuberculosis disease process;
— Medications, dosage, length of time given, and side effects (refer to Chapter 5);
— How to handle medication side effect;
— How to call nurse or physician;
— How to get emergency assistance;
— How to obtain medications;
— When to return to clinic for follow-up.

Medication Teaching Plan:
— Medications are usually taken as prescribed by a self-directed adherent patient;
— Medications can be taken daily or two or three times a week under the supervision of a community nurse or a board of health nurse. This is termed "directly observed intermittent therapy"(DOIT);
— Memory joggers, such as a calendar or drug box, are used to help establish habit of taking medications. Patients at high risk for forgetting to do so are alcoholics, psychiatric patients, and those with memory problems;
— Patients on antituberculosis medications for prophylaxis or for treatment of active disease must be assessed on a monthly basis;
— Teach side effects of medications.

Adjuncts To Teaching:
— Pamphlet on tuberculosis;
— Written instructions on medications, dosage, side effects;
— Post-test to measure patient's understanding if appropriate.

REFERENCES

Amin, N. M. (1994). Tuberculin skin testing. *Postgraduate Medicine*, *95(4)*, 46–56.

Avey, A. (1993, September). TB skin testing: How to do it right. *American Journal of Nursing*, *93 (9)*, 42–44.

Black, J. & Matassarin-Jacobs, E. (1993). *Medical-surgical nursing*: A psychophysiologic approach. Philadelphia: Saunders.

Centers for Disease Control. (1994). Guidelines for preventing the transmission of *Mycobacterium tuberculosis* in health-care facilities, 1994. *Morbidity and Mortality Weekly Report*, *43* (RR-13), 1–133.

Daugherty, J., Hutton, M., & Simone, P. (1993). Prevention and control of tuberculosis in the 1990s. *Nursing Clinics of North America, 28 (3)*, 599–611.

Huebner, R., Schein, M., & Bass, J. (1993). The tuberculin skin test. *Clinical Infectious Diseases*, 17, 968–975.

MacGregor, R. R. (1993). Tuberculosis: From history to current management. *Seminars in Roentgenology, XXVIII*, 101–108.

Roberts, G. D., & Thompson, G. P. (1994). Bacteriology and bacteriologic diagnosis of tuberculosis. In D. Schlossberg (Ed). *Tuberculosis* (3rd ed), (pp. 51–61), New York: Springer-Verlag.

Werhane, M.J., Snukst-Torbeck, G., & Schraufnagel, D.E. (1989). The tuberculosis clinic. *Chest*, *96*, 815–818

World Congress on Tuberculosis Program and Abstracts. (1992, November 16–19). Bethesda, Maryland.

7

ADHERENCE TO THE TUBERCULOSIS TREATMENT PLAN

Esther Sumartojo

The course of TB is affected by a number of factors, including the provision of adequate treatment, the infrastructure of health services for tuberculosis (TB), and patient adherence to medication regimens. Drug resistance can develop when medical treatment is inadequate or when patients do not adhere to an adequate regimen. Once drug resistance has developed in a particular patient, that drug-resistant disease may be passed on to other persons. Therefore, the quality of patient adherence has serious implications for the health of the public as well as the patient. Evidence suggests that physician practices (Sumartojo, Hale, & Geiter 1993) and the public health infrastructure (Brudney & Dobkin, 1991a) may in some situations be inadequate for treating TB. For many complex reasons, patients often fail to complete prescribed regimens for TB (Sumartojo, 1993). This chapter describes the problem of poor patient adherence, ways of measuring adherence, factors found to affect adherence, and findings from research on patient adherence to medication for TB and suggests approaches for improving adherence.

THE PROBLEM OF POOR PATIENT ADHERENCE

Adherence may be defined differently for various diseases. For TB it refers to patients taking medication as prescribed for the prevention of tuberculous infection or the treatment of active disease. The word adherence, used here as an alternative to the word compliance, is meant to avoid the incorrect connotation that the patient is submissive, subservient to the provider, and not able or willing to act independently of medical recommendations.

The problem of poor patient adherence to medical recommendations is not unique to TB. Hippocrates warned of it: "Keep a watch also on the faults of the patients, which often make them lie about the taking of things prescribed" (DiMatteo & DiNicola, 1982). One review (Haynes, Taylor, & Sackett, 1979) concluded that approximately 50% of patients fail to adhere to prescribed treatment for long-term illness. The Centers for Disease Control and Prevention (Centers for Disease Control and Prevention, 1992) estimates that approximately one-third of patients fail to complete preventive therapy for tuberculous infection for the prescribed 6 months, and one-fourth of patients for whom medication was prescribed for active tuberculosis fail to complete treatment within 1 year. In one clinical trial, approximately 50% of participants were nonadherent (Combs, O'Brien, Geiter, & Snider, 1987); in another, only one-fifth of patients were adherent by the 12th month of the study (Centers for Disease Control and Prevention, unpublished data). Researchers have found nonadherence to be as high as 90% among some patients being treated for TB (Brudney & Dobkin, 1991b; Werhane, Snukst-Torbeck, & Schraufnagel, 1989).

MEASURING PATIENT ADHERENCE

There are both direct and indirect ways to measure patient adherence. Direct ways include the measurement of the drug or its metabolite in blood or urine. Indirect ways include self-report; pill or container counts; special pill packaging devices; prescription refills and pharmacy records; and appointment keeping. Although improvement of symptoms, radiographic improvement, and conversion of sputum specimens to negative are sometimes used and might appear to be reliable means of measuring adherence, other factors can affect these such as drug-resistance of the organism or partial rather than full adherence to therapy (Snider & Hutton, 1989).

Direct Methods in TB

Urine assays can be used to identify antituberculosis medications (Burkhardt & Nel, 1980). Rifampin (RIF) is easily identified because it turns urine, feces, saliva, sweat, and tears red-orange. Isoniazid (INH) can be identified through simple chemical analysis or by using paper test strips (Henderson, 1986; Schraufnagel, Stoner, Whiting, Snukst-Torbeck, & Werhane, 1990; Snider et al., 1989) Urine assays can only estimate adherence because they are influenced by the rate at which patients metabolize the drugs. They may show a positive result even if the medication has not been taken regularly. Moreover, patients occasionally refuse to provide urine samples for testing.

Patient Self-Report

Patient self-report as a measure of adherence is subject to such variables as forgetfulness, reluctance to admit not taking medications, or fear of the health care provider (Sumartojo, 1993). One researcher showed that 28% of TB patients incorrectly reported taking medication as prescribed (Preston & Miller, 1964). Nevertheless, there is some evidence that patients with various medical conditions who have had some experience with a regimen can predict their own level of adherence (Kaplan & Simon, 1990) and that careful questioning by providers may yield accurate patient reports (Steele, Jackson, & Gutmann, 1990; Stewart, 1987). One report concluded that self-report is an acceptable measure of adherence if patients have agreed with providers to share the responsibility for treatment (Barnhoorn & Adriaanse, 1992).

Other Indirect Measures of Adherence

Indirect estimates of adherence are commonly used in TB clinics. These include pill counts, records of appointment keeping, and pharmacy or clinic records of whether and when patients picked up medications. However, if patients wish to appear adherent, they may discard medications or attend the clinic but still fail to take medications. Microelectronic devices have been used to record when and how often TB pills were taken from a box or bottle (Moulding, Onstad, & Sbarbaro, 1970; Cheung et al., 1988). These devices may be destroyed, lost, left open by patients who find them difficult to use, or they may be opened frequently by patients who are curious about how they work (Centers for Disease Control and Prevention, unpublished data). Additional research will assess the usefulness of medication monitors.

PREDICTING ADHERENCE

Health care providers are often unable to predict whether a particular patient will adhere to medical recommendations (DiMatteo et al., 1982). For example, research conducted in a general medical clinic indicated that physicians' predictions of nonadherence were accurate in fewer than 50% of cases (Mushlin & Appel, 1977). In a study of TB patients, physicians predicted nonadherence for only 32% of nonadherent patients; they also predicted nonadherence for 8% of adherent patients (Wardman, Knox, Muers, & Page, 1988). Often health care providers do not know that a patient is not following recommendations; many providers, unaware of the general problem of nonadherence, are not alert to the possibility of poor adherence (DiMatteo et al., 1982). Patients can go to great lengths to disguise nonadherence. Brenner and Pozsik (1993) give an example of a mother who poured out her child's medication each day, so that the amount of medication remaining matched what would be expected, but did not administer the medication to the child.

Nevertheless, providers would like to have a strategy for determining at the onset of treatment whether a particular patient will be adherent. However, in attempting to predict adherence, providers must consider environmental, structural, and operational aspects of the program that influence adherence but are beyond the patient's control. Adherence problems should not be attributed exclusively to patients; such attributions may bias providers against certain kinds of patients or prevent them from making provider-controlled changes to improve the quality of health care services.

Factors affecting adherence include those relating to

- The disease and treatment regimen;
- Features of the health care setting;
- The patient's, family and life circumstances; and
- The relationship between the patient and health-care provider.

A detailed discussion is beyond the scope of this chapter. The interested reader is referred to Snider et al. (1989).

Patient and Family Factors

Patient sociodemographic factors such as age, gender, race, ethnicity, occupation, income, and education tend to be inconsistent as predictors of adherence (Haynes, 1976; Kirscht & Rosenstock, 1979). Research has not shown a reliable relationship between adherence to TB medication and age (Alcabes, et al., 1989; Armstrong & Pringle, 1984; Barnhoorn & Adriaanse, 1992; Bell & Yach, 1988) or gender (Armstrong & Pringle, 1984; Barnhoorn et al., 1992; Bell & Yach, 1988; Henderson, 1984). Low family income (Barnhoorn et al., 1992; Buri, Vathesatogkit, Charoenpan, Kiatboonsri, & Buranaratchada, 1985; Corcoran, 1986;) and low educational level (Alcabes et al., 1989; Armstrong et al., 1984; Corcoran, 1986) are more consistent predictors of poor adherence, but these socioeconomic variables may be markers for other factors that are influencing adherence. For example, a lack of education or financial resources may relate to poor knowledge of, or access to, health care. Studies have found better adherence among patients with stronger family or social support (Barnhoorn et al., 1992; Corcoran, 1986; Nazar-Stewart, & Nolan, 1992; Sumartojo, 1992), more accurate knowledge about TB (Alcabes et al., 1989; Barnhoorn et al., 1992; Menzies, Rocher, & Vissandjee, 1993), greater concern about the seriousness of their condition (Alcabes et al., 1989; Barnhoorn & Adriaanse, 1992; Sumartojo, 1992), and better adherence early in TB treatment (Dubanoski, 1988; Menzies et al., 1993). Many anecdotal reports from providers attribute poor adherence to drug or alcohol abuse by patients.

It appears that patients who succeed in completing therapy believe that they have the support of family members and the physician or other health-care providers. These patients also believe that their own tuberculosis or tuberculous infection is a health problem that must be taken seriously. Their knowledge about TB and its treatment is more accurate. Additional studies of factors that predict adherence should inspire research on the effectiveness of interventions to improve adherence.

IMPROVING ADHERENCE: STRATEGIES AND APPROACHES

There is no simple approach to solving the multifaceted problem of poor adherence. Nurses and other providers should become familiar with the many issues involved, keep an open mind, respond to the characteristics and individual needs of the patients that they serve, and be innovative and persistent. The available information on adherence offers perspec-

TABLE 7.1 Improving the Quality of Interaction with the Patient

1. Create a partnership or an alliance with the patient.
2. Ask patients whether they are taking TB drugs; don't assume they are.
3. Give patient adequate time at each visit.
4. Don't frighten or intimidate the patient; be positive.
5. Get verbal and written commitments from the patient (Meichenbaum & Turk, 1987; Cuneo & Snider, 1989).
6. Treat the person, not just the disease.

tives, but few clear instructions, on how to improve patient adherence. The following suggestions are offered, drawn from various sources on TB and adherence (American Lung Association of South Carolina, 1989; Centers for Disease Control and Prevention, 1993; Cuneo & Snider, 1989; DiMatteo & DiNicola, 1982; Meichenbaum & Turk, 1987; Snider et al., 1989; Sumartojo, 1993).

Several interventions hold the potential to improve adherence. DiMatteo et al. (1982) recommend that the provider develop a partnership with the patient and help the patient remember to take medications. A partnership requires the provider to (1) communicate clearly so that the patient can understand, (2) avoid subtle cues of criticism of the patient's behavior, (3) be open-minded about the patient's beliefs and cultural norms, (4) accept the patient's frame of reference and avoid imposing on the patient the provider's own values about medical treatment, (5) understand and fulfill the patient's expectations about treatment, (6) reduce as much as possible the social distance between the provider and patient created by social or cultural differences, (7) recognize and address the patient's fears about his or her illness, and (8) treat the patient with dignity and respect.

Because people tend to forget and to underreport events relating to their health, providers should encourage patients to discuss their experiences with poor adherence or barriers to adherence. Providers should ask for specific information, such as how often the patient took medication or what doses were taken. The provider should also give clear feedback by listening carefully to what the patient says and by giving the patient positive verbal reinforcement for recalling specific adherence behaviors. The provider should ask the patient to make a commitment to remember and report adherence behaviors. As DiMatteo et al. (1982) point out, enhancing the patient-provider partnership and patient recall in these ways will improve patient reporting and will also improve patient adherence (see Table 7.1).

The patient must be included in the treatment process, and he or she

TABLE 7.2 Improving Adherence Through Treatment Approaches

1. Schedule the initial appointment soon after diagnosis.
2. Use appointment reminders.
3. Follow up quickly on missed appointments.
4. Tailor the regimen to the patient's needs; allow the patient some options.
5. Keep the regimen as simple as possible.
6. Give clear instructions concerning side effects.
7. Assess adherence early in treatment and try different strategies if needed.
8. Determine barriers to adherence; offer enablers to assist the patient.
9. Offer incentives, such as social or health care services.
10. Involve the family or social support system in treatment.
11. Ensure good case management practices.
12. Supervise therapy in accordance with CDC recommendations (Centers for Disease Control and Prevention, 1993).

should assume partial responsiblity for ensuring a positive outcome. Even though the patient is not responsible for becoming infected or sick with TB, he or she is responsible for making independent decisions about self-medication. The provider must do everything possible to educate, support, and persuade the patient to complete treatment, and to communicate information the patient can understand. Some TB patients do not appear capable of taking this kind of responsibility for their health, but it is likely that most are able to do so. Adherence can be improved by various treatment approaches (see Table 7.2).

Patient Education

Patient education has been used in combination with other interventions (Morisky et al., 1990; Seetha, Srikantaramu, Aneja, & Singh, 1981; Sower, & Breckenridge-Potterf, 1991; Wobeser, To, & Hoeppner, 1989), but its independent effect has not been measured. However, for other diseases, education alone has not been shown to be particularly successful in improving adherence. The best educational interventions instruct patients in ways of changing behavior, rather than simply providing information about the diagnosis or the disease (Meichenbaum et al., 1987).

Prochaska and DiClemente's Stages of Change Model (1992) suggests an important approach to community and patient education. The model states that people go through distinct stages of learning when they make a major change in behavior, such as taking medication every day. To be meaningful, educational information must be appropriate for each person's level of knowledge and his or her motivation to change. For exam-

TABLE 7.3 Improving Adherence Through Patient Education

1. Give vital information first in the patient interview.
2. Be concise and clear with instructions; the patient may be anxious after hearing the diagnosis.
3. Be clear from the start about the length of the regimen.
4. Avoid jargon. Don't overload the patient with too much information at one time.
5. Use educational materials that are culturally and linguistically appropriate for the patient.
6. Be alert that the patient may not be literate.
7. If using a translator, be sure he or she is familiar with the patient's culture.
8. Assess the patient's beliefs about TB; consider these beliefs when devising the treatment plan.
9. Review instructions; quiz the patient to ensure that he or she understands.
10. Describe the specific adherence behaviors required.
11. Clarify the patient's questions and respond clearly.
12. Give written instructions.

ple, persons who are at risk for TB may not be aware of, or concerned about, the need for a skin test. They may be influenced only by highly persuasive public messages that are designed to influence people in their own social group. Only when they are concerned about TB will they be interested in more specific information such as how to obtain a skin test. This model suggests that the provider inform patients that they may have difficulty adhering to the treatment regimen and help them devise strategies to deal with relapses. The Stages of Change Model assumes that people are most likely to pay attention to information when it is relevant to their needs and that they do not make major behavioral changes, such as taking daily medication, all at once, but in stages. Some ways of improving adherence through patient education are summarized in Table 7.3.

Cultural Beliefs

Research has addressed the influence of culturally determined beliefs about, and knowledge of, adherence to TB treatment (Rubel & Garro, 1992; Sumartojo, 1993). Data collected by CDC in an ethnographic study of minority and foreign-born TB patients and persons from the patients' communities indicate strong and specific beliefs about TB (Centers for Disease Control, unpublished data). The data suggest that these beliefs, influenced by group and cultural norms, hinder persons from seeking screening or adhering to preventive therapy, leading to the con-

TABLE 7.4 Clinic Operations That Improve Adherence

1. Ensure a physical environment that is acceptable to patients.
2. Ensure that all staff behave in a positive manner towards patients.
3. Ensure that schedules and practices are tailored to the patients' needs.
4. Ensure that records management, pharmacy, and lab services are efficient and do not inconvenience patients.
5. Nurture staff morale; provide training as needed.

clusion that programs must tailor services to the distinct beliefs, attitudes, and concerns about TB in their communities.

Directly Observed Therapy

Directly observed, or supervised, therapy (DOT) means that a health care worker observes the patient taking his or her medication and is recommended as an effective method for ensuring adherence (Centers for Disease Control and Prevention, 1993; Pozsik, 1993; Weis, Slocum, Blais, King, Nunn, Matney et al., 1994). Strategies for delivering DOT include having patients go to the TB clinic or health care provider to take medications; having community health or outreach workers go to the patient's home or arrange to meet with the patient; having a school nurse, employee nurse, prison guard, clerk at a homeless shelter, or some other designated person administer medication to the patient. Acceptable intermittent medication regimens make DOT more feasible. DOT should be presented so that patients perceive it as positive, not punitive. For example, patients can share in some decisions, such as the best place to receive DOT. Providers should ensure that nonprofessional persons delivering DOT are trained and monitored. It is essential that providers ensure the individual rights of patients by tailoring DOT to patients' particular needs and circumstances. DOT is labor intensive. In addition, it demands the careful organization and management of the community workers or persons responsible for delivering medication, and it requires a positive alliance between the provider and the patient so that the patient will attend the clinic or be available at another place to receive medication. The CDC has stated that "DOT should be considered for all patients because of the difficulty in predicting which patients will adhere to a prescribed treatment regimen" (Centers for Disease Control and Prevention, 1993, p.6). Even directly observed therapy is not foolproof. Pozsik in a section subtitled "dirty tricks" discusses methods patients may use to avoid taking medication even with DOT. These include not swallowing pills, holding pills in their mouth, spitting pills out into opaque cups, and even inducing vomiting after the nurse or health care worker leaves the room (Pozsik, 1993).

Community health workers, or outreach workers, not only supervise therapy, but they also follow the course of treatment and support and assist patients in many ways. In some TB programs, volunteer community health workers have assisted in TB elimination activities (Manalo, Tan, Sbarbaro, & Iseman, 1990; Nuyangulu, Nkhoma, & Salaniponi, 1990; Westaway, 1988;). Typically, these workers are from the patients' own communities. To be successful, programs must adequately train and supervise the workers. These workers must be respected in the communities they serve (Westaway, 1988).

Other Strategies

DOT is not a panacea for the problem of increasing TB; rather, it is one strategy of an effective health care service. Typically, DOT is part of a program of services that also includes individualized case management; enablers to help patients overcome barriers to adherence; clinic practices that make services accessible and acceptable for patients; staff who are skilled at working with the groups served by the treatment center; and additional health or social services for patients. Table 7.4 suggests ways that clinic operations can be structured to improve adherence. Good patient services, a strong health care infrastructure, and a good relationship between the patient and the provider are also integral to controlling and preventing TB. Treatment outcomes depend on many factors: (1) the personal and social characteristics of patients and of the staff who work at TB clinics, (2) the culturally determined knowledge and beliefs of patients and staff, (3) the quality of interaction between patients and providers, (4) the quality of health services provided by the TB treatment center and the quality of the health care infrastructure that supports the treatment center, (5) the quality of public and patient information about TB, (6) the quality of training that the health-care professional providers and staff have received, and (7) more distant factors such as the economy, law, and politics.

Effective treatment strategies have included the use of drug injections (Sbarbaro, 1979) and special packaging using blister calendar packs (Valeza & McDougall, 1990). Incentives (such as money or birthday cakes) and enablers (such as bus tokens or food) have been used to improve adherence (American Lung Association of South Carolina, 1989; Morisky et al., 1990; Snider et al., 1989), but little systematic research has been carried out to assess their effects. Some interventions provide social incentives (e.g., by agreeing to take medication, patients make a social contract with the provider and may derive an emotional reward from completing the agreement). One study found that patients who made both verbal and written commitments to return to have their tuberculin skin test reactions read were more likely to return (Wurtele, Galanos, & Roberts, 1980), and another described a successful "breakfast club" for alcoholic patients (Edwards, 1988). Family involvement in adherence activities has also improved adherence (Seetha, et al., 1981). Social rewards may be more powerful motivators for adherence than material incentives.

Some TB treatment centers offer what might be called comprehensive services because they take a holistic view of the patient's needs and use an assortment of methods to address adherence. For example, one report describes a successful program with multiple approaches: (1) clinics were held at times and places that were found to be convenient according to surveys of patients and community leaders; (2) appointment schedules were used to reduce waiting time for patients; (3) persons needing social services were appropriately referred; (4) nurses made home visits to patients who missed appointments; (5) community groups and health department personnel were educated about the need for the specialized services; and (6) efforts were made to develop medical teams that worked well together and held positive views of the patients (Curry, 1968). Other effective comprehensive programs have put together well-integrated health teams and coordinated community resources (McAdam, Brickner, Scharer, Crocco, & Duff, 1990), and provided incentives or enablers such as food, transportation, or additional medical services (McDonald, Memon, & Reichman, 1982). One successful clinic (Werhane et al., 1989) employed a pulmonary nurse specialist and a nurse epidemiologist, who fostered strong relationships with patients and provided careful case management, scheduled appointments, appointment reminders, and the close follow-up of missed appointments. Patients were given money for transportation and referred for assistance with social, financial, and other medical problems as needed. Treatment was simplified by the use of combination tablets.

In general, comprehensive services are effective because they include health teams of personnel who assume responsibility for providing continuity of care and careful case management and follow-up, make the clinic accessible and acceptable to patients, create a system for providing social services to patients, and offer short-course treatment regimens that include supervised therapy. This kind of service has been shown to improve treatment success among patients who might otherwise fail to complete treatment (McDonald et al., 1982). Using a comprehensive approach, the provider or treatment center takes responsibility for treatment outcomes and seeks the participation of patients by offering them the assistance they need (Etkind, Boutotte, Ford, Singleton & Nardell, 1991). Several publications include additional recommendations for improving patient adherence to TB treatment (American Lung Association of South Carolina, 1989; Cuneo, et al., 1989; Snider, et at., 1989). Providers and program personnel are urged to consider these sources and other relevant information, such as studies of treatment approaches and incentives found in the research literature, to develop strategies relevant to their patients that take into account local conditions and environment.

SUMMARY

Nonadherence to the treatment plan has been and continues to be a problem for treatment of TB. Indeed, it is one of the major reasons for the continuing spread of drug-susceptible and drug-resistant TB. Because they provide much of the care to TB patients, nurses have a vital role to play in improving patient adherence to planned TB therapy. Many of the recommended strategies in this chapter should be familiar as good nursing care practices. Successful TB nurses will draw upon their own knowledge as well as research findings of the kind reviewed here to ensure positive treatment outcomes for their patients.

REFERENCES

Alcabes, P., Vossenas, P., Cohen, R., Braslow, C., Michaels, D., & Zoloth, S. (1989). Compliance with isoniazid prophylaxis in jail. *American Review of Respiratory Disease, 140*, 1194–1197.

American Lung Association of South Carolina (1989). *Enablers and incentives* (booklet). Columbia, SC: Author.

Armstrong, R. H., & Pringle, D. (1984). Compliance with anti-tuberculous chemotherapy in Harare City. *The Central African Journal of Medicine, 30*, 144–148.

Barnhoorn, F., & Adriaanse, H. (1992). In search of factors responsible for noncompliance among tuberculosis patients in Wardha District, India. *Social Science and Medicine, 34*, 291–306.

Bell, J., & Yach, D. (1988). Tuberculosis patient compliance in the Western Cape, 1984. *South African Medical Journal*, *73*, 31–33.

Brenner, E., & Pozsik C. (1993). Case holding. *Lung Biology in Health and Disease*, *66*, 183–205.

Brudney, K., & Dobkin, J. (1991a). A tale of two cities: tuberculosis control in Nicaragua and New York City. *Seminars in Respiratory Infections*, *6*, 261–272.

Brudney, K., & Dobkin, J. (1991b). Resurgent tuberculosis in New York City. *American Review of Respiratory Disease*, *144*, 745–749.

Buri, P. S., Vathesatogkit, P., Charoenpan, P., Kiatboonsri, S., & Buranaratchada, S. (1985). A clinic model for a better tuberculosis treatment outcome and factors influencing compliance. *Journal of the Medical Association of Thailand*, *68*, 356–360.

Burkhardt, K. R., & Nel, E. E. (1980). Monitoring regularity of drug intake in tuberculous patients by means of simple urine tests. *South African Medical Journal*, *57*, 981–985.

Centers for Disease Control and Prevention (1992). Management of persons exposed to multidrug-resistant tuberculosis. *Morbidity and Mortality Weekly Report*, *41*, 59–71.

Centers for Disease Control and Prevention (1993). Initial therapy for tuberculosis in the era of multidrug resistance: Recommendations of the Advisory Council for the Elimination of Tuberculosis. *Morbidity and Mortality Weekly Report, 42(No.RR–7)* , 1–8.

Cheung, R., Dickins, J., Nicholson, P. W., Thomas, A. S. C., Smith, H. H., Larson, H. E., Deshmukh, A. A., Dobbs, R. J. & Dobbs, S. M. (1988). Compliance with anti-tuberculous therapy: A field trial of a pill-box with a concealed electronic recording device. *European Journal of Clinical Pharmacology*, *35*, 401–407.

Combs, D., O'Brien, L. J., Geiter, L. J., & Snider, D. E. (1987). Compliance with tuberculosis regimens: Results from USPHS Therapy Trial 21. *American Review of Respiratory Disease*, *135*, A138. (Abstract)

Corcoran, R. (1986). Compliance with chemotherapy for tuberculosis. *Irish Medical Journal*, *79*, 87–90.

Cuneo, W. D., & Snider, D. E. (1989). Enhancing patient compliance with tuberculosis therapy. *Clinics in Chest Medicine*, *10*, 375–380.

Curry, F. J. (1968). Neighborhood clinics for more effective outpatient treatment of tuberculosis. *The New England Journal of Medicine*, *279*, 1262–1267.

DiMatteo, M. R., & DiNicola, D. D. (1982). *Achieving patient compliance: The psychology of the medical practitioner's role*. New York: Pergamon Press.

Dubanoski, J. P. (1988). Preventive health behavior: A model of adherence prediction. *Dissertation Abstracts International*, *48*, 3152.

Edwards, B. B. (1988). The breakfast club. *The Florida Nurse*, *36*, 9.

Etkind, S., Boutotte, J., Ford, J., Singleton, L., & Nardell, E. A. (1991). Treating hard to treat tuberculosis patients in Massachusetts. *Seminars in Respiratory Infections*, *6*, 273–282.

Haynes, R. B. (1976). A critical review of the "determinants" of patient compliance with therapeutic regimens. In D. L. Sackett & R. B. Haynes (Eds.), *Compliance with Therapeutic Regimens* (pp.26–39). Baltimore: The Johns Hopkins University Press.

Haynes, R. B., Taylor, D. W. & Sackett, D. L. (Eds.), (1979). *Compliance in health care*. Baltimore: The Johns Hopkins University Press.

Henderson, M. A (1984). Tuberculosis in a developing country: Experience of the TB service at BMH, Dharan. *Journal of the Royal Medical Corps, 130*, 22–30.

Henderson, W. T. (1986). The development and use of the Potts-Cozart tube test for the detection of isoniazid (INH) metabolites in urine. *Journal of the Arkansas Medical Society, 82*, 445–446.

Kaplan, R. M., & Simon, H. J. (1990). Compliance in medical care: reconsideration of self-predictions. *Annals of Behavioral Medicine, 12*, 66–71.

Kirscht, J. P., & Rosenstock, I. M. (1979). Patients' problems in following recommendations of health experts. In G. C. Stone, F. Cohen & N. E. Adler (Eds.), *Health Psychology: A Handbook* (pp. 189–215). San Francisco: Jossey-Bass.

Manalo, F., Tan, F., Sbarbaro, J. A., & Iseman, M. D. (1990). Community-based short-course treatment of pulmonary tuberculosis in a developing nation. *American Review of Respiratory Disease, 142*, 1301–1305.

McAdam, J. M., Brickner, P. W., Scharer, L. L., Crocco, J. A., & Duff, A. E. (1990). The spectrum of tuberculosis in a New York City men's shelter clinic (1982–1988). *Chest, 97*, 798–805.

McDonald, R. J., Memon, A. M. &, Reichman, L. B. (1982). Successful supervised ambulatory management of tuberculosis treatment failures. *Annals of Internal Medicine, 96*, 297–302.

Meichenbaum, D., & Turk, D. C. (1987). *Facilitating treatment adherence: a practitioner's guidebook*. New York: Plenum Press.

Menzies, R., Rocher, I., & Vissandjee, B. (1993). Factors associated with compliance in treatment of tuberculosis. *Tubercule and Lung Disease, 74*, 32–37.

Morisky, D. E., Malotte, C. K., Choi, P., Davidson, P., Rigler, S., Sugland, B., & Langer, M. (1990). A patient education program to improve adherence rates with antituberculosis drug regimens. *Health Education Quarterly, 17*, 253–267.

Moulding, T., Onstad, G. D., & Sbarbaro, J. A. (1970). Supervision of outpatient drug therapy with the medication monitor. *Annals of Internal Medicine, 73*, 559–564.

Mushlin, A. I., & Appel, F. A. (1977). Diagnosing potential noncompliance. *Archives of Internal Medicine, 137*, 318–321.

Nazar-Stewart, V., & Nolan, C. M. (1992). Results of a directly observed intermittent isoniazid preventive therapy program in a shelter for homeless men. *American Review of Respiratory Disease, 146*, 57–60.

Nuyangulu, D. S., Nkhoma, W. N., & Salaniponi, F. M. L. (1990). Factors contributing to a successful tuberculosis control programme in Malawi.

Bulletin of the International Union Against Tuberculosis, *66* (Supplement), 45–46.

Pozsik, C.J. (1993). Compliance with tuberculosis therapy. *Medical Clinics of North America*, *77(6)*, 1289–1301.

Preston, D. F., & Miller, F. L. (1964). The tuberculosis outpatient's defection from therapy. *The American Journal of the Medical Sciences*, *247*, 55–58.

Prochaska, J. O., & DiClemente, C. C. (1992). Stages of change in the modification of problem behaviors. In M. Hersen, R. M. Eisler, & P. M. Miller (Eds.), *Progress in Behavior Modification* (pp. 184–218). Sycamore, IL: Sycamore.

Rubel, A. J., & Garro, L. C. (1992). Social and cultural factors in the successful control of tuberculosis. *Public Health Reports*, *107*, 626–636.

Sbarbaro, J. A. (1979). Compliance: Inducements and enforcements. *Chest*, *76* (Suppl.), 750–756.

Schraufnagel, D. E., Stoner, R., Whiting, E., Snukst-Torbeck, G., & Werhane, M. J. (1990). Testing for isoniazid: An evaluation of the Arkansas method. *Chest*, *98*, 314–316.

Seetha, M. A., Srikantaramu, N., Aneja, K. S., & Singh, H. (1981). Influence of motivation of patients and their family members on the drug collection by patients. *The Indian Journal of Tuberculosis*, *XXVIII*, 182–190.

Snider, D. E., & Hutton, M. D. (1989). *Improving patient compliance in tuberculosis treatment programs*. Atlanta: CDC, Public Health Service, U.S. Department of Health and Human Services.

Sower, P., & Breckenridge-Potterf, S. (1991). Utah Department of Health: Refugee tuberculosis education program. *TB Notes, Spring*, 7. (Published by the Division of Tuberculosis Elimination, National Center for Prevention Services, Centers for Disease Control and Prevention).

Steele, D. J., Jackson, T. C., & Gutmann, M. C. (1990). Have you been taking your pills? The adherence-monitoring sequence in the medical interview. *Journal of Family Practice*, *30*, 294–299.

Stewart, M. (1987). The validity of an interview to assess a patient's drug taking. *American Journal of Preventive Medicine*, *3*, 95–100.

Sumartojo, E. (1992). A psychosocial approach to predicting adherence among tuberculosis patients. *American Review of Respiratory Disease*, *145 (pt. 2, No.4, supp)*, A818. (Abstract).

Sumartojo, E. (1993). When TB treatment fails: A social behavioral account of patient adherence. *American Review of Respiratory Disease*, *147*, 1311–1320.

Sumartojo, E., Hale, B.E., & Geiter, L. (1993). Physician practices in preventing and treating tuberculosis: Results of a national survey. *American Review of Respiratory Disease*, *147 (No. 4, pt. 2, supp)*, A722. (Abstract).

Valeza, F. S. & McDougall, A. C. (1990). Blister calendar packs for treatment of tuberculosis. *Lancet*, *335*, 473.

Wardman, A. G., Knox, A. J., Muers, M. F., & Page, R. L. (1988). Profiles of non-compliance with antituberculous therapy. *British Journal of Diseases of the Chest*, *82*, 285–289.

Weis, S., Slocum, P. C., Blais, F. X., King, B., Nunn, M., Matney, G. B.,

Gomez E., & Foresman, B. H. (1994). The effect of directly observed therapy on the rates of drug resistance and relapse in tuberculosis. *New England Journal of Medicine, 330,* 1179–1184.

Werhane, M. J., Snukst-Torbeck, G., & Schraufnagel, D. E. (1989). The tuberculosis clinic. *Chest, 96,* 815–818.

Westaway, M. S. (1988). *Compliance with tuberculosis treatment: The role of the voluntary health worker.* Report for the Tuberculosis Research Institute of the Medical Research Council, Republic of South Africa.

Wobeser, W., To, T., & Hoeppner, V. H. (1989). The outcome of chemoprophylaxis on tuberculosis prevention in the Canadian Plains Indian. *Clinical and Investigative Medicine, 12,* 149–153.

Wurtele, S. K., Galanos, A. N., & Roberts, M. C. (1980). Increasing return compliance in a tuberculosis detection drive. *Journal of Behavioral Medicine, 3,* 311–318.

PART III
Prevention

8

SCREENING FOR TUBERCULOSIS: AN IMPORTANT PREVENTION TOOL

Carol D. Harriman and Felissa L. Cohen

Screening, tuberculin skin testing, early diagnosis of active disease, and prompt tracing and screening of contacts of persons with recently diagnosed pulmonary TB are all ways of preventing the spread of TB. Such TB control programs have been a traditional component of public health agencies because people with transmissible TB pose a potential health threat to their communities until they have completed adequate treatment. This chapter will describe screening and tuberculin skin testing.

SCREENING PROGRAMS

Currently, the principal reasons for conducting TB screening programs are to identify persons with

TABLE 8.1 Classification of Persons Exposed to and/or Infected With *M. tuberculosis*

Classi-fication	Expos-ure	TB Skin Test	Bacteri-ology	Clinical Symptoms	Radio-graphy	Preventive Therapy
0. No tuberculosis exposure, not infected	No	Negative	Negative	No	Negative	No
1. Tuberculosis exposure, no evidence of infection	Yes	Negative	Negative	No	Negative	Considered
2. Tuberculosis infection, no disease	Yes	Positive	Negative	No	Negative	Considered
3. Tuberculosis clinically active	Yes	Usually Positive	Positive/ Negative	Yes/No	Positive/ Negative	No
4. Tuberculosis not clinically active	Yes	Positive	Negative	No	Negative for current disease/ Positive, stable	Considered
5. Tuberculosis suspect (diagnosis pending) (3 mos. only)	Yes/No	Positive/ Negative	Positive/ Negative	Yes/No	Positive/ Negative	No

1. Tuberculous infection at high risk of developing tuberculosis who would benefit from preventive therapy, and
2. Those with tuberculosis who need treatment.

Other reasons for which screening activities might reasonably be carried out include: 1) assessing the extent and trends of the TB in a given population or area; 2) evaluating the appropriateness of TB screening programs; and 3) increasing public awareness about TB. As described below, the standard screening tool for tuberculous infection in high risk populations is the tuberculin skin test using the Mantoux method, which is described in detail later in this chapter (Centers for Disease Control, 1990). When the object of a screening program is to identify individuals with existing pulmonary tuberculosis rather than tuberculous infection, health care providers may elect to use chest radiography (x-ray) and/or sputum smear examinations instead, although such approaches may be more costly. There is also some debate over whether or not routine chest radiographs in well populations (such as preemployment screening) are useful when no symptoms or positive tuberculin reaction is present (Lanphear & Snider, 1991). However, they may be useful (and cost effective) for those who may not return for readings of their skin test, such as those who are transients (Centers for Disease Control, 1990).

All screening programs must be coupled with educational efforts with provisions made for follow-up, diagnostic testing, and therapy if indicated. Tracing and investigation of the contacts of those persons ultimately found to have active TB is essential in the prevention of the spread of TB and is discussed in Chapter 10. After testing and diagnosis, for the purposes of public health programs, persons exposed to and/or infected with *M. tuberculosis* may be classified operationally as shown in Table 8-1.

For Whom Is Tuberculin Testing Indicated?

The CDC have made recommendations about screening including the conducting of tuberculin skin testing programs in various populations. In the report detailing the plan for the elimination of TB in the United States, the CDC (1989c) recommend that by 1991, all United States residents have the results of at least one tuberculin skin test documented in their medical record. Needless to say, those who have positive or significant test results should be evaluated with regard to their risk of developing tuberculosis, and appropriate action taken. The CDC recommend initial, two-step testing at the time of employment for health care workers. Those who are nonreactive should undergo repeat testing at times commensurate with that institution's risk assessment (see Chapter 9) at intervals that may range from every 3 months in high-risk areas to every year in low-risk areas. These apply to staffs of such facilities as TB clinics, mycobacteriology laboratories, shelters for the homeless, nursing homes, substance-abuse treatment centers, dialysis units, correctional institutions, hospitals, mental institutions and home health care agencies (Centers for Disease Control, 1994).

Although it is important to identify high-priority groups for screening by means of tuberculin testing, flexibility must also be maintained. In other words, some of those groups that are now high priority may subsequently decline in risk, and others who are not now considered high-priority groups may become at higher risk (Centers for Disease Control, 1990b).

TABLE 8.2 Persons in Whom Tuberculin Skin Testing is Indicated

---

- Persons with signs, symptoms (cough, hemoptysis, weight loss, etc.) and /or laboratory abnormalities (e.g., radiographic abnormality) suggestive of clinically active TB.

- Recent contacts of persons known to have or suspected of having clinically active TB.

- Persons with HIV infection.

- Persons with abnormal chest roentgenograms compatible with past TB.

- Persons with other medical conditions that increase the risk of TB (silicosis, injecting drug use, diabetes mellitus, prolonged corticosteroid therapy, immuno-suppressive therapy, some hematologic and reticuloendothelial diseases, end-stage renal disease, and clinical situations associated with rapid weight loss).

- Groups at high risk of recent infection with *M. tuberculosis*, such as immigrants from Asia, Africa, Latin America, and Oceania; medically underserved populations; personnel and long-term residents in some hospitals, nursing homes, mental institutions, and correctional facilities.

Source: American Thoracic Society (1992), Control of Tuberculosis in the United States. *American Review of Respiratory Disease, 146,* 1628.

Those considered to be at higher risk than the general population and for whom tuberculin skin testing is indicated are listed in Table 8.2. The rationale for most of these persons is evident. Further explanation for some was reviewed in Chapter 3 or is discussed later. The development of screening programs and sites should be done based on risk. Thus the CDC recommend that tuberculin testing for persons with HIV-infection should be conducted at the following sites in addition to TB or chest disease clinics:

- substance abuse treatment centers;
- AIDS clinics;
- HIV counseling and testing sites;

- sexually transmitted disease clinics; and
- other facilities in which HIV testing is offered (Centers for Disease Control, 1990b).

Prisons and Jails. Poor ventilation and overcrowding in prisons may promote the transmission of infection from persons with undiagnosed TB to inmates, staff, and visitors. Frequent transfers, both within and between prisons, also contribute to the spread of TB within the prison system. Given the above situation, the CDC recommends skin testing of inmates on entry and annually for persons who are skin-test negative. Persons who are skin test positive or who have symptoms of tuberculosis should have chest x-rays within 3 days of admission. Inmates who are HIV-positive should receive chest x-rays regardless of tuberculin test outcome. Jails pose a special problem in TB screening because large numbers of detainees pass through them relatively quickly. For this reason, the CDC (1989a) recommends tuberculin skin test screening only for those with stays greater than 7 days. Persons with symptoms of active tuberculosis, regardless of length of incarceration, should receive prompt chest x-rays and acid-fast bacilli (AFB) sputum studies. Some jails have shifted to screening by chest radiographs (Skolnick, 1993).

Medically Underserved Low-Income Populations. As discussed elsewhere, the more frequent occurrence of TB is related to lower socioeconomic status, leading to crowded living conditions or lack of shelter, poorer access to health care, lack of transportation, and so on. Occupational groups that include a higher percentage of low-income persons include unskilled laborers, migrant farm workers, lower paid health-care workers and food handlers. Special efforts may be needed to screen such occupational groups at their work site or homesites (Centers for Disease Control, 1990b). For example, TB testing can be advertised and carried out at migrant camps; however if the migrant worker is relocated before the tests can be read, they will be lost to follow-up. A means of longer term follow-up, such as a tracking network, has been suggested (Richard, 1994).

It is important to involve community groups in efforts to reach underserved and minority populations. In some cases locally based community organizations can conduct screening with the assistance of health departments, and in others health departments can coordinate such efforts with other groups including private and public agencies, health-care providers, community groups and others. Coalitions of such groups can advise the community in the best ways to conduct screening programs and provide treatment, services, and education (Centers for Disease Control, 1992).

TUBERCULIN TESTING

Tuberculin skin testing is used to detect whether or not a person is infected with *M. tuberculosis*; it does not tell whether or not active disease is present. Two types of materials are used in this country for tuberculin testing. These preparations are Old Tuberculin (OT) and Purified Protein Derivative (PPD). OT is a filtrate prepared from sterilized concentrates of *M. tuberculosis* that is used with multiple puncture testing devices, and PPD is a precipitate prepared from OT that is used with either multiple puncture testing devices or intradermally via the Mantoux test (American Thoracic Society, 1990; Lordi & Reichman, 1994).

Multiple Puncture Test

The percutaneous multiple puncture test (Heaf® or Tine® test) has been used generally in low-risk populations for general screening; it should not be used in tuberculin testing surveillance programs or in high-risk groups. Its use today is limited. In the multiple puncture test, tuberculin is introduced either by puncture through a film of liquid tuberculin or by puncture with an applicator whose points are coated with dry tuberculin. These tests use either concentrated OT or PPD, but the amount cannot be precisely controlled and, therefore, these tests are not diagnostic. Reactions are measured at 48 to 72 hours and 1) if discrete papules are seen, the diameter of the largest single papule should be measured; 2) if there is a coalescence of papular reactions, the largest diameter of coalescent induration should be measured; and 3) if the reaction is vesicular, it is recorded as positive. Only vesicular reactions are considered positive. Other reactions should be verified by use of the Mantoux test described below. Multiple puncture tests should not be used in serial testing or surveillance programs, which are discussed later in this chapter (American Thoracic Society, 1990).

Mantoux Test

It is generally accepted that the Mantoux test is the standard and best method for identifying individuals infected with tuberculosis (Centers for Disease Control, 1990). The basic principle underlying a reaction to the Mantoux test is that of delayed hypersensitivity (Lordi & Reichman, 1994). Persons who have been infected with *M. tuberculosis* or other mycobacteria and who have normal, intact cell-mediated immunity will have a positive reaction to the Mantoux test between 48 and 72 hours

TABLE 8.3 Mantoux Test Procedure

---

1. The patient should be seated comfortably. The inner (dorsal) aspect of the forearm, about 4 inches below the elbow (usually the left) is the preferred site, but any red, swollen, or abraded areas should be avoided, as should areas with visible veins (Avey, 1993).

2. Using a 1/4-to 1/2-inch, 26-or 27-gauge needle with the bevel and needle opening facing upward, the test is administered by the slow intradermal injection of exactly 5 tuberculin units (TU) (0.1 milliliters) of PPD just under the skin. This should be done by holding the skin of the forearm tautly and inserting the needle at a 10-to 15-degree angle without aspirating. Usually, the needle tip can be seen through the skin (Amin, 1994).

3. A distinct, pale, tense wheal (similar to a mosquito bite) of approximately 6 to 10 millimeters should appear. The needle should be quickly withdrawn, and the site should not be massaged after needle withdrawl (Smith & Duell, 1992; Timby, 1989). There should be no leakage.

4. If this does not happen, a valid test has not been administered, and another should be repeated immediately at another site at least 2 inches from the first (Centers for Disease Control, 1989).

5. Charting should include the date and time the test was done; the name, strength, manufacturer, and lot number of the injected antigen; the dose administered; the arm used; the specific site of administration; the reason for testing; and the signature of the person who administered the test. The reason for testing should be included in the entry because the information will be essential in making the correct interpretation of the test result.

---

after administration as discussed below. This reaction occurs as a result of the sensitization of certain lymphocytes in response to infection with mycobacteria and exposure to these antigens, causing the lymphocytes to recognize the antigen and respond (American Thoracic Society, 1990).

Test Material and Administration. PPD (discussed above) is the usual test material used for the Mantoux test. PPD is available in multidose vials containing either 10 or 50 doses. Special care is needed for the storage of PPD used for the test. It should be stored in a darkened refrigerator because loss of potency occurs with exposure to light and contamination. Heat speeds the rate of bacterial growth within the solution once the vial has been opened. Tuberculin has the tendency to adhere to the insides of glass and plastic syringes, but the addition of Tween® (a detergent) has helped to prevent this. Nonetheless, the vial of PPD should be removed from the refrigerator only when the Mantoux test is about to be administered, the dose promptly drawn up using meticulous aseptic technique, the vial returned immediately to the darkened refriger-

TABLE 8.4 Reading the Mantoux Test

1. Typically readings are done 48 to 72 hours after testing when reactions are maximal (American Thoracic Society, 1990).

2. Readings should be made in good light with the forearm supported on a firm surface and slightly flexed at the elbow (Centers for Disease Control, 1989a).

3. The basis of reading is the presence or absence of induration (not erythema or redness) which may be initially located visually (from a side view against the light as well as by direct light) and then defined by palpation. The borders of the induration can be marked with a pen or felt marker and then measured using a flexible ruler calibrated in millimeters, which is placed directly on the skin over the reaction's widest diameter in the transverse axis (see Figure 8.1).

4. The size of the reaction is recorded in the patient's chart—in millimeters of induration as measured across the transverse diameter—along with the date and time it was read and the reader's signature. When there is no induration, *0 millimeters* should be recorded. Failure to record the result of a Mantoux test in millimeters of induration may result in unnecessary repeat skin testing. Words such as "positive" or "negative" and "significant" or "insignificant" should not be used in recording results (Centers for Disease Control, 1989a). They are interpretations rather than clinical observations.

ator, and the dose administered without delay (American Thoracic Society, 1981; Bass, 1993). The procedure for this test is shown in Table 8.3.

Reaction and Reading. After administration of the Mantoux test, the typical delayed hypersensitivity reaction normally begins about 5 to 6 hours after administration, reaches a maximum at about 48 to 72 hours (the optimal period for reading), and subsides slowly over a period of days. In some persons immediate hypersensitivity, beginning shortly after administration, may be observed to either the tuberculin or other components of the fluid. These are infrequent and usually disappear within 24 hours. A few persons may show vesicular or ulcerating local reactions that can be accompanied by lymphadenitits, lymphangitis, lymphadenopathy and fever (American Thoracic Society, 1990). Correct reading of the Mantoux test is very important. Components of the reading are shown in Table 8.4, and a reactive test is illustrated in Figure 8.1.

Interpretation. What is known about an individual's medical conditions and that person's known or estimated risk of past exposure to contagious tuberculosis disease determines which of three cut points will be used for interpretation (American Thoracic Society, 1990; Centers for Disease

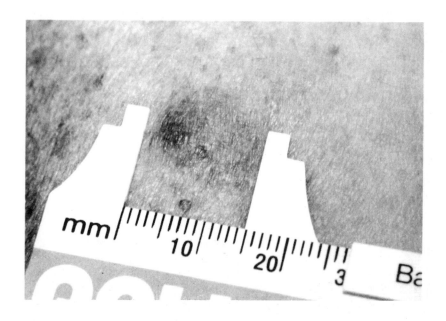

FIGURE 8.1 A reactive Mantoux test. Note that it is the area of induration, not the area of erythema, that is measured and recorded.

Control, 1989b). The major cut-off points are 5 or more, 10 or more, and 15 or more milliliters of induration. Five millimeters or more is considered positive for the highest risk groups who may have immuno-suppression because of their own disease, having a limited ability to react to tuberculin, even if infected with *M. tuberculosis*; and for those who have had close contact with a person with tuberculosis or have chest radiographs consistent with inactive tuberculosis. Ten or more milliliters is considered positive for persons not meeting the previous criteria but who have other known risk factors for tuberculosis. This category also includes employees in hospitals, mycobacterial laboratories and other high-risk exposure settings. Fifteen or more millimeters of induration is considered positive for persons with no risk factors for tuberculosis. These categories are shown in Figure 8.2. For each of the categories, reactions below the cutting point are considered negative (American Thoracic Society, 1990; Centers for Disease Control and Prevention, 1994; Huebner, Schein, & Bass, 1993). CDC have defined interpretation for recent converters on the basis of both induration and age as follows:

5 or more millimeters induration is considered positive for the highest risk groups, such as:

- Persons with HIV infection;

- Persons who have had close contact with an infectious tuberculosis case;

- Persons who have chest radiographs consistent with old, healed tuberculosis;

- Intravenous drug users whose HIV status is unknown.

10 or more millimeters induration is considered positive for other high risk groups, such as:

- Foreign-born persons from high prevalence areas (such as Asia, Africa, and Latin America);

- Intravenous drug users known to be HIV seronegative;

- Medically-underserved low income populations, including high-risk racial or ethnic minority populations (especially blacks, Hispanics, and Native Americans);

- Residents of long-term care facilities (such as correctional institutions, nursing homes, mental institutions);

- Persons with medical conditions which have been reported to increase the risk of tuberculosis such as silicosis, being 10 percent or more below ideal body weight, chronic renal failure, diabetes mellitus, high dose corticosteroid and other immunosuppresive therapy, some hematologic disorders (such as leukemias and lymphomas), and other malignancies;

- Locally identified high risk populations;

- Children who are in one of the high risk groups listed above; and

- Health care workers who provide services to any of the high risk groups.

15 or more millimeters induration is considered positive for persons with no risk factors for tuberculosis.

Negative Reactions - For each of the categories, reactions below the cutting point are considered negative.

FIGURE 8.2 Mantoux test Interpretation.

Source: Centers for Disease Control, Mantoux tuberculin skin test reading wall chart (00-5564), 1989.

TABLE 8.5 Factors Causing Decreased Ability to Respond to Tuberculin

Factors Related to the Person Being Tested
   Infections
      —Viral (measles, mumps, chicken pox)
      —Bacterial (typhoid fever, brucellosis, typhus, leprosy, pertussis, overwhelming
         tuberculosis, tuberculous pleurisy)
      —Fungal (South American blastomycosis)
   Live virus vaccinations (measles, mumps, polio)
   Metabolic derangements (chronic renal failure)
   Nutritional factors (severe protein depletion)
   Diseases affecting lymphoid organs (Hodgkin's disease, lymphoma, chronic lymph-
   ocytic leukemia, sarcoidosis)
   Drugs (corticosteroids and many other immunosuppressive agents)
   Age (newborns, elderly patients with "waned" sensitivity)
   Recent or overwhelming infection with *M. tuberculosis*
   Stress (surgery, burns, mental illness, graft versus host reactions)

Factors Related to the Tuberculin Used
   Improper storage (exposure to light and heat)
   Improper dilutions
   Chemical denaturation
   Contamination
   Adsorption (partially controlled by adding Tween® 80)

Factors Related to the Method of Administration
   Injection of too little antigen
   Delayed administration after drawing into syringe
   Injection too close

Factors Related to Reading the Test and Recording Results
   Inexperienced reader
   Conscious or unconscious bias
   Error in recording

Source: American Thoracic Society (1990). Diagnostic standards and classification of
tuberculosis. *American Review of Respiratory Disease, 142*, p. 732.

a 10 millimeter or greater increase within a 2-year period is classifed as
a conversion for persons less than 35 years of age and a 15 mm or more
increase within a 2-year period is classified as a conversion for persons
35 years of age and older (Centers for Disease Control and Prevention,
1994). A 5mm or more increase in persons who meet the criteria listed
under 5 or more mm in Figure 8.2 is considered a conversion by some.
   Some researchers have questioned whether groups with a high prevalence of anergy such as those who are injecting drug users or HIV-

infected should have a 2 mm induration cutoff (Graham, Nelson, & Solomon, 1992), but others believe that routine chest radiographs are necessary in such groups in order not to miss those with active TB (Bellin, Fletcher, & Safyer, 1993). Persons who have received Bacille Calmette-Guérin (BCG) vaccination (see Chapter 5) in the past often react to tuberculin. The current recommendation is that large reactions on the Mantoux test, partiularly in those from countries with a high tuberculosis prevalence, should not be considered as being due to the BCG vaccination, but that the person should be evaluated for the presence of TB.

Those who have small or no reactions may be genuinely free from tuberculous infection, or there may be another reason such as conditions that impair delayed hypersensitivity, leading to a false negative reaction. These situations may be related to the person being tested, the material used, the method of interpretation, or the test reading and result recording and are summarized in Table 8.5. Anergy is one of these and is considered below. Persons who are very ill with disseminated TB may not react to the tuberculin skin test (Huebner, et al., 1993).

What does a significant or positive reaction to a Mantoux test mean? It means that hypersensitivity to mycobacteria has developed. It does not specify that it is *M. tuberculosis* because there can be cross-reaction to antigens from other mycobacteria (Bass, 1993). In general, the larger the reaction, the more likely that the sensitivity is to *M. tuberculosis* rather than some other type of mycobacteria. The significant reaction to the Mantoux skin test does not necessarily mean that tuberculosis infection is present. For example, false positive reactions can occur if the person is infected with a nontuberculous mycobacteria, such as *M. kansaii* or has had a previous BCG vaccination (Glassroth, 1993; Huebner, et al., 1993). Further diagnostic efforts (sputum smear examination and culture and chest radiograph in the case of pulmonary TB) are needed to make such a determination.

The timing of conversion can be important if tuberculin testing is conducted periodically in populations of persons exposed to TB who are tuberculin negative such as nurses on medical units. This is discussed below.

The Booster Phenomenon and Serial Testing

The booster effect or recall phenomenon is based on the waning of delayed-type hypersensitivity (DTH) over time and its recall by a subsequent tuberculin skin test. Repeated tuberculin skin testing in persons who do not have tuberculous infection will not sensitize them to tubercu-

TABLE 8.6 Summary of Guidelines for Anergy Testing

1. All persons with HIV infection should receive a PPD-tuberculin skin test (5TU,PPD by Mantoux method).

2. Because of the occurence of anergy to PPD among persons with HIV infection at risk of tuberculosis, persons with HIV infection should also be evaluated for DTH anergy at the time of PPD testing.

3. Companion testing with two DTH* antigens (*Candida*, mumps, or tetanus toxoid) administered by the Mantoux method is recommended. However, a multipuncture device, with administers a battery of DTH antigens, may be used.

4. Any induration to a DTH antigen, measured at 48 hours to 72 hours, is considered evidence of DTH responsiveness; failure to elicit a response is considered evidence of anergy.

5. Those persons with a positive ($\geq$5mm in duration) PPD reaction are considered to be infected with *M. tuberculosis* and should be evaluated for isoniazid preventive therapy after active tuberculosis has been excluded.

6. Persons who manifest a DTH response but have a negative PPD reaction are, in general, considered not to be infected with *M. tuberculosis*

7. Anergic, tuberculin-negative persons whose risk of tuberculous infection is estimated to be $\geq$10% should also be considered for isoniazid preventive therapy after active tuberculosis is excluded.

8. Although CD4 counts should be performed as part of the evaluation and management of persons with HIV infection, this measurement is not a substitute for anergy evaluation.

*delayed hypersensitivity

Source: Centers for Disease Control (1991). Purified protein derivative (PPD)-tuberculin anergy and HIV infection: Guidelines for anergy testing and management of anergic persons at risk of tuberculosis. *Morbidity and Mortality Weekly Report*, *40*(RR-5), p. 33.

lin. However, in those who have had DTH due to any mycobacterial infection or to BCG vaccination (see Chapter 5), a waning of the reaction over time may occur. This may result in tuberculin skin test reactions that are negative. A subsequent test done at least 1 week later may then result in an increase in the reaction size because it recalls the past infection. In other words, sometimes the immune system fails to react to tuberculin testing because it has temporarily "forgotten" that it was once invaded by an antigen that is similar to tuberculin, and its ability to react to that antigen has waned over the years. The test, although failing to elicit an initial positive reaction, often will stimulate the immune system into a responsive mode. In summary, if after an initial tuberculin test, a second test is administered after at least 1 week and as long as 1 year or more later, the infected person will generally respond with a clearly positive reaction. This is called the "booster phenomenon." The first test "boosted" the immune system into responsiveness. The second test elicited a positive reaction. The booster effect increases in age and is most frequently seen in those 55 years of age and older (American Thoracic Society, 1990).

The booster phenomenon can make it difficult to distinguish those who are newly infected from those who are not. It is important to determine whether the booster effect is caused by tuberculous infection or not, and if it is, whether this infection is recent or not. If an infected individual requires two tests to elicit a reaction and the interval between the two tests is long, a boosted response may be misinterpreted. Thus, the infected person may have remained unidentified as such for a year or more, and when discovered, may receive an incorrect preventive therapy recommendation based on the misperception that the person is a converter rather than a reactor.

Serial testing often on a regular annual or more frequent basis depending upon risk assessment has been recommended for staff in locations and institutions such as nursing homes, hospitals, long-term care facilities, HIV clinics, mycobacterial laboratories, dialysis units, and units where pentamidine is administered and for residents of nursing homes on admission (Centers for Disease Control and Prevention, 1994) (see Chapter 9). Therefore it may be appropriate for the initial baseline testing to be a two-step process in which a second tuberculin test is given 1 or 2 weeks after the first. In this manner, those who do not boost after 1 or 2 weeks, but have reactive tests after 1 year can be presumed to have newly acquired tuberculous infection and can be treated appropriately (American Thoracic Society, 1990; Centers for Disease Control, 1989a,b; Thompson, Glassroth, Snider, & Farer, 1979).

Recent Conversion

Recent tuberculin skin test converters are considered to be a high-risk group. The CDC has classified an increase of induration of 10 or more mm within a 2-year period as a conversion among persons below 35 years of age, an increase of 15 or more mm within a 2-year period as a conversion for persons 35 years of age or older (Centers for Disease Control and Prevention, 1994), and 5 or more mm under certain circumstances.

Anergy

Persons who are immunosuppressed, particularly those who have HIV-infection, often have anergy (the inability to mount an immune response) to delayed-type hypersensitivity reactions (DTH). Therefore, the CDC have recommended that persons with HIV-infection, even if asymptomatic, should be evaluated for delayed-type hypersensitivity anergy in conjunction with PPD testing. The CDC also recommend consideration of anergy testing for those in risk groups for both tuberculous and HIV infection (Centers for Disease Control, 1991). For example, there is a high prevalence of anergy among injecting drug users and those who have rapid weight loss for various reasons (Zoloth et al., 1993). Other conditions may also result in anergy, either on a temporary or permanent basis. These include alcoholism, theraputic ultraviolet light exposure, and pernicious anemia (Pesanti, 1994).

Companion testing with two delayed-type hypersensitivity skin-test antigens are recommended, typically, mumps antigen, tetanus toxoid, and perhaps *Candida* antigen, as well as others such as *Trichophyton* may be included, and a Multitest anergy panel preparation is used by many (Pesanti, 1994). Testing is given concurrently with the tuberculin Mantoux. Those persons with a positive DTH response (induration of any amount) to one or more of the DTH antigens but who do not respond to the tuberculin test are not considered to be infected with *M. tuberculosis*. Those who do not respond to DTH testing are considered to be anergic. Those reactions of more than 2 mm of induration to any of the skin tests including tuberculin are not considered anergic (Centers for Disease Control, 1991; Centers for Disease Control and Prevention, 1994). A summary of guidelines for anergy testing are shown in Table 8.6.

After Tuberculin Testing

Persons who are found to have reactive tuberculin skin tests must receive the appropriate diagnostic testing and, if indicated, preventive therapy or medical treatment. These are discussed below and in Chapters 4 and 5.

SUMMARY

Screening programs are a useful public health approach in the detection of those with tuberculous infection or tuberculosis. Such programs usually employ tuberculin skin testing (ideally the Mantoux test) but may use chest radiography or sputum smear examination under certain circumstances. The interpretation of tuberculin skin test reactions is based on the assessed risk for TB in the person being tested. Appropriate follow-up of persons with reactive tuberculin skin tests regarding diagnosis, preventive or other therapy, contact tracing, and education are essential.

REFERENCES

American Thoracic Society. (1990). Diagnostic standards and classification of tuberculosis. *American Review of Respiratory Disease, 142*, 725–735.

American Thoracic Society. (1981). The tuberculin skin test. *American Review of Respiratory Disease, 124*, 356–363.

Amin, N. M. (1994). Tuberculin skin testing. *Postgraduate Medicine, 95(4)*, 46–56.

Avey, M. A. (1993). TB skin testing: How to do it right. *American Journal of Nursing, 93(9)*, 42–44.

Bass, J. B. Jr. (1993). The tuberculin test. *Lung Biology in Health and Disease, 66*, 139–148.

Bellin, E., Fletcher, D., & Safyer, S. (1993). Abnormal chest x-rays in intravenous drug users: Implications for tuberculosis screening programs. *Americal Journal of Public Health, 83*, 698–700.

Centers for Disease Control. (1989a). Screening for tuberculosis: Administering and reading the Mantoux Test. Videotape 0260–CPS.

Centers for Disease Control. (1989b). A strategic plan for the elimination of tuberculosis in the United States. *Morbidity and Mortality Weekly Report, 38* (S–3).

Centers for Disease Control. (1990). Screening for tuberculosis and tuberculous infection in high-risk populations. *Morbidity and Mortality Weekly Report, 39(RR–8)*, 1–7.

Centers for Disease Control. (1991). Purified protein derivative (PPD)-tuberculin anergy and HIV infection: Guidelines for anergy testing and management of anergic persons at risk of tuberculosis. *Morbidity and Mortality Weekly Report, 40* (RR–5), 27–33.

Centers for Disease Control. (1992). Prevention and control of tuberculosis in U.S. communities with at risk minority populations: Recommendations of the Advisory Committee For Elimination of Tuberculosis. *Morbidity and Mortality Weekly Report, 41* (RR–5), 1–11.

Centers for Disease Control. (1994). Guidelines for preventing the transmission of *Mycobacterium tuberculosis* in health-care facilities, 1994. *Morbidity and Mortality Weekly Report, 43* (RR-13), 1–133.

Glassroth, J. (1993). Diagnosis of tuberculosis. *Lung Biology in Health and Disease, 66,* 149–165.

Graham, N. M. H., Nelson, K. E., Solomon, L. et al. (1992). Prevalence of tuberculin positivity and skin test anergy in HIV-1-seropositive and-seronegative intravenous drug users. *Journal of the American Medical Association, 267,* 369–373.

Lordi, G. M. & Reichman, L. B. (1994). Tuberculin skin testing. In D. Schlossberg (Ed). *Tuberculosis* (3rd ed), (pp. 63–68), New York: Springer-Verlag.

Pesanti, E. L. (1994). The negative tuberculin test. *American Journal of Respiratory and Critical Care Medicine, 149,* 1699–1709.

Richard, J. R. (1994). TB in migrant farmworkers. *Journal of the American Medical Association, 271,* 905.

Skolnick, A. A. (1993). Correction facility TB rates soar: Some jails bring back chest roentgenograms. *Journal of the American Medical Association, 268,* 3175–3176.

Smith, S. F., & Duell, D. J. (1992) *Clinical nursing skills,* 3rd ed., Norwalk, CT, Appleton & Lange.

Thompson, N. J., Glassroth, J. L., Snider, D.E. Jr., & Farer, L. S. (1979). The booster phenomenon in serial tuberculin testing. *American Review of Respiratory Disease, 119,* 587–597.

Timby, B. K. (1989). *Clinical nursing procedures,* Philadelphia: Lippincott.

Zoloth, S. R., Safyer, S., Rosen, J., Michaels, D., Alcabes, P., Bellin, E., & Braslow, C. (1993). Anergy compromises screening for tuberculosis in high-risk populations. *American Journal of Public Health, 83,* 749–751.

9

PREVENTING THE SPREAD OF TUBERCULOSIS IN HEALTH-CARE FACILITIES AND HOME HEALTH CARE

Joan E. Otten

An effective infection control program in health-care facilities is necessary to prevent the transmission of *Mycobacterium tuberculosis* from patient to patient, to health-care workers, and to visitors. Such a program requires early detection (including surveillance), isolation, and treatment of persons with active TB, and any TB control plan should emphasize achieving these (Centers for Disease Control and Prevention, 1993). This must include the availability of proper equipment and education of the health-care workers regarding TB so that the necessary, appropriate infection-control precautions may be taken. The strategies and resultant tuberculosis policies and procedures are based on principles that can be applied regardless of the health care setting. This includes the home health care setting, as described later in the chapter. Depending on the situation, there may always be some level of risk to health care workers of exposure to a patient with active TB, but this risk can be reduced. The keys to lowering exposure risk are 1) a high index of suspicion for TB in order to identify cases rapidly; 2) the prompt and proper implementation of infection control measures; and 3) appropriate TB education and training for health care workers.

The recent reports of outbreaks of multidrug-resistant TB (MDR-TB) in hospitals and prisons have been studied by the Centers for Disease Control and Prevention (CDC) as well as the facilities experiencing the outbreak. Two major factors are thought to have contributed to these outbreaks in hospitals. These were delay in the diagnosis of TB, and delay in instituting appropriate infection control measures. Patients were not being properly isolated when they were infectious (Centers for Disease Control, 1991). When adequate control measures are in place, such outbreaks can often be prevented.

The most comprehensive documents describing transmission precaution measures are available from the CDC (1994) and the American Thoracic Society (1992). The CDC have have published recommendations for facilities providing long-term care to the elderly (Center for Disease Control; 1990b) (see Chapter 11) and for correctional institutions (1989). The challenge facing each health-care facility is to implement these recommendations in order to provide a safe working environment. The CDC guidelines prioritize numerous prevention measures and have attempted to place them in a hierarchical order of priority in order to aid the facility. These include

- Administrative measures to reduce the risk of exposure to persons with infectious TB. Included are the development and implementation of effective written policies and protocols for the rapid detection, isolation, diagnosis, and treatment of persons suspected of having TB, and implementation of effective staff work practices;

- Engineering controls to prevent the spread and reduce concentration of infectious droplet nuclei. This includes local exhaust ventilation, preventing air contamination in areas adjacent to the infectious source case, general ventilation to dilute and remove contaminated air and air filtration or ultraviolet light germicidal irradiation (UVGI) to clean the air; and

- Use of personal respiratory protective equipment in situations in which exposure to infectious TB may occur, such as in rooms where patients with known or suspected TB are isolated and in treatment rooms for such patients (Centers for Disease Control and Prevention, 1994).

Each will be described in more detail below.

ADMINISTRATIVE MEASURES

Within a health-care facility, it is usually the infection control committee that has the responsibility and authority to implement TB control measures, determine the risk of exposure to health care workers within the facility, and monitor for outbreaks. If it is determined that there may be a danger to patients or staff, the members of the committee must take corrective action. A major goal of the committee is to prevent nosocomial transmission to health care workers, other patients, and visitors. A risk assessment of the institution is one way to use information to design and formulate policies and should be done for the general facility and for special areas such as pulmonary clinics, emergency departments, and others (Centers for Disease Control and Prevention, 1993). Aspects to be assessed in determining policies for institutions meeting minimal, very low, intermediate, and high-risk situations are shown in Figure 9.1. The TB control plan for the institution should be based on the risk assessment and responsibility should be assigned for its implementation and enforcement (Centers for Disease Control and Prevention, 1994). An optimum TB control program for all health care facilities is shown in Table 9.1. Selected aspects of it are discussed in more detail in the rest of this chapter. Any TB program must be continually evaluated for adherence and effectiveness and redesigned if necessary according to the evaluation results.

IDENTIFICATION OF PATIENTS WITH TB

The most important step in preventing the transmission of TB is the rapid identification of the patient who is either known to have, or is suspected of having, active infectious TB. Once recognized, the patient can then be placed on isolation with implementation of the appropriate infection control precautions as discussed later in this chapter. In order to accomplish this, the person who has the first contact with the patient—be it in the emergency department, clinic, or home setting—must be aware of the prevalence of TB in the population served by the health care facility and must be alert for the common signs and symptoms of TB as discussed in Chapter 4 (productive cough, fever, anorexia, fatigue, night sweats,

(continued, p. 162)

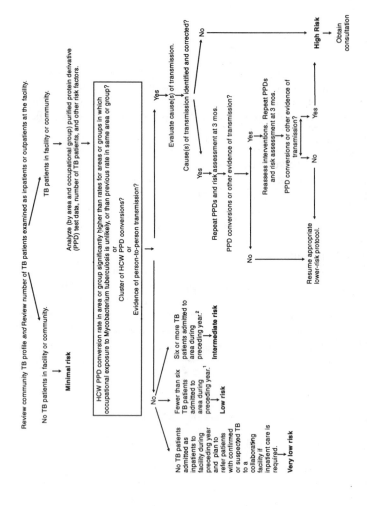

FIGURE 9.1 Risk assessment for developing a TB control plan.

[1]For occupational groups, exposure to fewer than 6 TB patients for HCWs during the preceding year.
[2]For occupational groups, exposure to 6 or more TB patients for HCWs during the preceding year.
Adapted from Centers for Disease Control and Prevention (1994). Guidelines for preventing the transmission of *Mycobacterium tuberculosis* in health-care facilities, 1994. *Morbidity and Mortality Weekly Report*, 43(No. RR-13), p. 10.

TABLES 9.1 Optimum TB Control Program for All Health-Care Facilities

I. Initial and Periodic Risk Assessment
   A. Evaluate health-care worker PPD test conversion data
   B. Determine TB prevalence among patients overall and in specific areas
   C. Repeat risk assessment at appropriate intervals
II. Written TB Infection Control Program
   A. Document all aspects of TB control
   B. Identify individual(s) responsible for TB control program
   C. Explain and emphasize hierarchy of controls
III. Implementation
   A. Assignment of Responsibility
      1. Assign responsibility for TB control program to individual(s)
      2. Ensure that persons with expertise in infection control, occupational health and engineering are identified and included
   B. Risk Assessment and Periodic Reassessment of the Program
      1. Select initial risk protocols
      2. Observe health-care worker infection control practices
      3. Repeat risk assessment at appropriate intervals
   C. Identification, Evaluation, and Treatment of Patients with TB
      1. Symptom screen for each patient:
         a. On initial encounter in emergency department or ambulatory care setting
         b. Before or at admission
      2. Radiologic and bacteriologic screening for patients with symptoms of TB
      3. Promptly initiate treatment
   D. Management of Outpatients With Possible Infectious TB
      1. Promptly initiate TB precautions
      2. Place patients in separate waiting areas or TB isolation rooms
      3. Give patients surgical mask, box of tissues, instructions
   E. Managing Inpatients Who Have Possible Infectious TB
      1. Prompt isolation and initiation of treatment for patients with suspected or known infectious TB
      2. Monitoring of response to treatment
      3. Follow appropriate criteria for discontinuation of isolation
   F. Engineering Recommendations
      1. Local exhaust and general ventilation should be designed in collaboration with persons with expertise in ventilation engineering
      2. In areas where infectious TB patients receive care, use single-pass system or recirculation after HEPA filtration
      3. Use additional measures, if needed, in areas where TB patients may receive care
      4. Design TB isolation rooms in health-care facilities to achieve ≥ 6 air changes per hour (ACH) for existing facilities and ≥ 12 ACH for new or renovated facilities
      5. Regularly monitor and maintain engineering controls
      6. TB isolation rooms that are being used should be monitored daily to ensure they maintain negative pressure relative to the hallway and all surrounding areas.
      7. Exhaust TB isolation room air to outside or, if unavoidable, recirculate after HEPA filtration
   G. Respiratory Protection
      1. Respiratory protective devices should meet recommended performance criteria

Table 9.1, continued

---
   2. Should be used by persons entering rooms in which patients with known or suspected infectious TB are being isolated, when performing cough-inducing or aerosol-generating procedures on such patients, and in other settings where administrative and engineering controls are not likely to protect them from inhaling infectious airborne droplet nuclei.

   3. A respiratory protection program is required where respiratory protection is used

H. Cough-inducing Procedures
   1. Should not be performed on TB patients unless absolutely necessary
   2. Should be performed using local exhaust or in individual TB isolation room
   3. After completion, TB patients should remain in booth or enclosure until cough subsides

I. TB Education
   1. All health-care workers should receive periodic education appropriate to their job
   2. Should include epidemiology of TB in the facility
   3. Should emphasize concepts of pathogenesis and occupational risk
   4. Should describe practices that reduce TB transmission

J. Health-care Workers Counseling and Screening
   1. Counsel all health-care workers regarding TB and tuberculous infection
   2. Counsel all health-care workers about increased risk if immunocompromised
   3. PPD test all health-care workers on employment and repeat at periodic intervals
   4. Screen symptomatic health-care workers for active TB

K. Evaluate health-care workers, PPD test conversions and possible nosocomial TB transmission

L. Coordinate efforts with public health department

Adapted from Centers for Disease Control. (1994). Guidelines for preventing the transmission of *Mycobacterium tuberculosis* in health-care facilities, 1994. *Morbidity and Mortality Weekly Report*, *43*(RR-13), 20–21.

weight loss, etc), or for clinical suspicion and know what to look for or what additional questions should be asked. This first contact person *must have the authority* to institute TB isolation based on his or her educated evaluation of the patient. It is of the utmost importance that these suspect TB patients (including pregnant women) are promptly and appropriately isolated in order to prevent transmission to persons within the institution. It is necessary to institute these isolation procedures before the results of the chest radiograph, tuberculin skin test, or acid-fast bacilli (AFB) smear are known. In areas such as ambulatory care areas, patients who have symptoms suggestive of TB should be placed in a separate waiting area, preferably in a room meeting TB isolation requirements, evaluated promptly, and should be given a surgical mask to put on (Centers for Disease Control and Prevention, 1994).

For patients who have a history of TB and are currently taking anti-TB medications, a determination must be made regarding the patient's adherence to the medication regimen. When there is a question of nonadherence, that patient should be placed in TB isolation. Patients with known or suspected multidrug-resistant TB should be isolated until determined to be both adherent and noninfectious (see Chapters 5 and 10).

HIV-Infected Patients

One of the greatest potential risks for transmission of TB within a health care setting are patients who are HIV-positive and present with undiagnosed pulmonary disease. Any HIV patient who is suspected of having *Pneumocystis carinii* pneumonia (PCP) must also be evaluated for the possibility of TB. In HIV-infection, TB can be manifested with minimal or atypical signs and symptoms along with a chest radiograph that can be normal or may indicate infiltrates or other findings. Therefore, if any suspicion exists, TB isolation should be instituted. HIV-infected patients, because of their immunosuppression, are vulnerable to infections from others and should not be exposed to persons with TB. Thus, clinics for those who are HIV infected or otherwise immunocompromised should not be in the same areas or on the same days or times as clinics seeing patients with active TB (Centers for Disease Control and Prevention, 1994). It is preferable to put patients with suspected or confirmed TB on oral prophylaxis for PCP if medically indicated instead of aerosolized pentamidine treatment.

Children

Children with suspected or confirmed primary TB should be evaluated for potential infectiousness. Young children with TB are less likely to be infectious than are adults. Although children with TB usually do not have a cough and do not produce sputum, the CDC are currently recommending that the following children be placed in TB isolation until they are determined to be noninfectious: those with pulmonary or laryngeal TB; those with a cough or who are undergoing cough-inducing procedures; and those who have a positive sputum AFB smear gastric aspirate, or pulmonary cavitation (Centers for Disease Control, 1994). A child with HIV infection who presents with pulmonary symptoms and infiltrates on chest x-ray should be evaluated for the need for isolation for suspected TB. Parents and visitors of any child with TB should be evaluated for signs and symptoms of active pulmonary or laryngeal TB (See Chapter 11). If such signs and symptoms are present, they should be excluded from visitation until they have been screened for active TB, treated if necessary, and determined to be non-infectious. In the case of the need for visitation prior to the work-up, the visitor must wear a surgical mask while in the health care facility.

Pregnancy

The pregnant woman with tuberculous infection or active TB must be appropriately identified, isolated, evaluated, and treated during pregnancy. The risk is actually greater to the newborn after delivery if there is contact with the mother who has infectious TB than it is to the fetus. When the pregnant woman is identified as having either tuberculous infection or active TB, there should be a contact investigation of household members and other close contacts with the appropriate medical follow-up and treatment prior to the newborn being discharged to that household. Chapter 10 discusses the contact investigation and Chapter 11 considers TB and pregnancy. Pregnant women with a prior history of a reactive tuberculin skin test or tuberculosis should be evaluated for active disease and treatment if warranted.

TB ISOLATION

Patients suspected or known to have active infectious TB (usually pulmonary or laryngeal) should be placed on TB isolation (also known as AFB isolation) which is more involved than respiratory isolation. There are three major reasons for TB isolation:

1. to separate persons who have confirmed or suspected infectious TB from other people;
2. to prevent escape of droplet nuclei into the halls and other areas of the health-care facility;
3. to provide an environment that lowers the concentration of droplet nuclei via engineering controls (Centers for Disease Control and Prevention, 1994).

Essentially, TB isolation entails placing patients in a private room with the door closed, specified ventilation characteristics, and the use of a respiratory protective device by anyone who enters the room. In the event that a room with proper air handling is not immediately available, the above procedures should still be implemented pending transfer to an isolation room. A sign must be placed on the door indicating the precautions that are necessary for all individuals entering the room but which may only say "Isolation" to protect the patient's privacy. In addition, the front of the patient's medical record must be labeled to indicate that the patient is on TB isolation. A personal respiratory protective device must be readily available to anyone entering the room. It is put on outside the room and then removed after leaving the room and closing the door. Gowns, gloves, and eye protection are to be worn as indicated for universal precautions. The number of people entering the room should be kept to a minimum.

When placed on TB isolation, patients should be taught about TB transmission and the reasons for isolation. This teaching should include how patients should cover their mouths and noses when sneezing or coughing as discussed in Chapter 6. The need for patients to stay in their room with the door closed should be emphasized, and every effort made to facilitate patient adherence including the use of incentives (See Chapter 7) (Centers for Disease Control and Prevention, 1994). Recreation or diversions should be provided to prevent boredom and/or depression. Since the main reason for isolation is to keep patients with active TB apart from others, diagnostic and treatment procedures should be carried out in their room when possible and transport through the health-care facility should be avoided. However, when the patient must leave the room because of a medical procedure that cannot be carried out within the room, a surgical mask that covers the patient's nose and mouth must be worn. The department that is to receive the patient must be notified in advance of the need for TB isolation so that personnel can protect themselves as well as conduct the test appropriately. Procedures should be conducted in a room with ventilation meeting TB isolation room requirements; waiting in the area should be minimized; and the procedure should be scheduled at times that are less busy to minimize contact with others. In general, elective operative procedures should be delayed until the patient is no longer infectious. If surgery must be done, it should be scheduled at the end of the day or at a time when there is a minimum number of staff and patients. Further precautions are detailed by CDC (Centers for Disease Control and Prevention, 1994).

During the medical work-up of the patient, TB isolation must continue to be carried out until the patient is determined to be noninfectious. It is not recommended that patients who share the same potential TB diagnosis also share a room because one or the other may not actually have TB. An order for a sputum smear or culture for AFB is a good indication that there is a suspicion of TB and, therefore, isolation is warranted. The determination for isolation should be made at this time and should not wait for the results of the AFB sputum smear. Even with a fast turn-around time for the smear results, there would be a delay in the implementation of isolation if the practice were not to isolate the patient until the results are known, and health care workers and other patients would be needlessly exposed to TB. When a tuberculin skin test is ordered, there must be a determination made as to whether the patient requires TB isolation. This decision is based upon the history of the patient for prior TB or exposure to TB and signs and symptoms of TB, as well as known factors that place the patient at high risk for TB as discussed in Chapters 3, 4, 5, and 8.

Cough-Inducing Procedures

The procedures during the medical work-up or treatment of any patient that can generate the most airborne droplet nuclei through stimulation of coughing are sputum collection, sputum induction, intubation, bronchoscopy, suctioning, and aerosol treatments such as pentamidine therapy for PCP. Other procedures can also generate aerosols, such as irrigation of abscesses caused by TB (Centers for Disease Control and Prevention, 1994). CDC (1994) recommend that procedures that induce coughing not be performed on patients with infectious TB unless absolutely necessary. If there is a question of active TB in a patient undergoing any of these procedures, TB isolation must be carried out. A specially designed, self-contained booth or chamber can be utilized in the outpatient setting to isolate the patient during these treatments. The air in the chamber must be at negative pressure in relation to the surrounding environment and is then filtered through high-efficiency particulate air (HEPA) filters before being returned to the room. These chambers must be part of the preventive maintenance program to assure proper functioning. The patient must remain isolated in the chamber and not returned to the waiting room until the coughing subsides.

ENGINEERING CONSIDERATIONS

As discussed earlier, engineering controls include ventilation in general and specific facility areas. The design system should meet federal, state, and local requirements. Air handling requirements for TB patient isolation rooms are described by such groups as the Health Resources and Services Administration (1984) and the CDC (Center for Disease Control 1994). Specifications require a minimum of six air exchanges per hour for isolation and treatment rooms; the direct exhaustion of air to the outside so that there is no re-circulation of the air to other areas of the facility, and negative pressure of the isolation room in respect to the corridor, so that air flows from the corridor into the isolation rooms and not vice-versa when the door is open. The most difficult aspect of maintaining appropriate air handling is keeping the isolation room at negative pressure. Negative pressure is created in a room when more air is exhausted than is supplied (Nicas, Sprinson, Royce, Harrison, & Macher, 1993). One way to determine that the desired negative pressure is correct is through the use of a smoke tube that generates "smoke" and indicates the direction of the flow of air. The "smoke" should be drawn into the room when the tube is placed at the bottom of the outside of the closed door of an isolation room, indicating the pressure is negative in relation to the corridor. If the "smoke" is blown out into the corridor, the pressure is positive. If there is no motion of the "smoke," the pressure is neutral. If a smoke tube is not available, another quick way to determine the flow of the air is to hold up a single sheet of paper tissue outside the room with the door slightly ajar.

Rooms that show positive pressure should not be used for TB isolation patients. The use of rooms with neutral pressure are not ideal, but if negative pressure rooms are unavailable, these neutral rooms provide more protection than the positive ones. The aim is to not have the airborne droplet nuclei generated by the TB patient blown out into the corridor and carried into other rooms or be circulated through the air handling system to other areas of the facility.

There have been numerous reports of the difficulty of maintaining a room at negative pressure. In a recent study of 121 rooms with negative pressure in seven midwestern hospitals, of the 115 tested by the investigators, 52 (45%) actually had positive pressure to the corridors with the doors closed (Fraser, et al., 1993). Several steps can be taken to assist with the maintenance of negative pressure, and these are described by Fraser and colleagues (1993). Some of the most important are keeping the doors and windows closed in the TB isolation room.

Ultraviolet Germicidal Irradiation (UVGI)

Another control measure to prevent the transmission of TB is upper room UVGI, which is a method of air disinfection that has been recommended as a supplement to other TB environmental control measures. Early studies done by Riley and associates (1962) showed that UV lamps were effective in disinfecting the air and preventing the transmission of TB to animals. It uses a narrow band of the ultraviolet part of the electromagnetic spectrum to inactivate airborne pathogens (Nardell, 1993, p. 1326). Placement of the UV fixtures is in the upper room, above people's heads, making it relatively safe for those in the lower room, providing the fixtures are properly designed and installed (Nardell, 1993; Riley, 1993). UVGI appears to be particularly useful as a supplement in isolation or treatment rooms, in corridors and in emergency department or outpatient waiting rooms where patients with TB are seen but may be unrecognized (Centers for Disease Control and Prevention, 1994). In New York and several other cities, a study is underway to determine the efficacy of UVGI in shelters for the homeless ("Ultraviolet faces revival . . . ", 1994).

Maintenance of the equipment is necessary. In addition, effects can include possible photosensitivity in those taking certain medications or who have certain medical conditions. It can also cause keratoconjunctivitis and erythema of the skin, and broad-spectrum UV irradiation has been associated with squamous and basal cell carcinomas of the skin (Centers for Disease Control and Prevention, 1994). In order to prevent harmful exposure to people, installation of UV lamps should be done by a qualified consultant, and there must be appropriate safety measures in place. These include signs advising people not to gaze directly at the UV lamps, advising them of the need to protect eyes and skin, and education of health care workers in the facility.

RESPIRATORY PROTECTION DEVICES

There have been many discussions by experts from CDC, National Institute for Occupational Safety and Health (NIOSH, 1981), Occupational Safety and Health Administration (OSHA) and medical staff experts regarding the respiratory protective device that should be used by healthcare workers entering the room of a TB isolated patient to protect themselves from inhaling droplet nuclei (U.S. Department of Health and Human Services, 1994). This protective device should filter out the tubercle bacillus, which is in the range of one to 5 microns, and the device should provide a good face seal so that the individual wearing it must breathe through the device instead of having the air, with the droplet nuclei, leak through gaps between the respirator and the face. These devices should be fluid resistant to meet the recommendations for universal precautions. A determination regarding the type of respiratory protective device to be used must take into consideration the requirement of the agency responsible for inspections concerning occupational exposure to TB within the health-care facility. In October 1993, OSHA issued a new enforcement policy directive requiring the use of a NIOSH approved high-efficiency particulate air (HEPA) respirator as the minimum acceptable level of respiratory protection.

A respiratory protective device is placed on the face to cover the mouth and nose and protects the wearer by removing the contaminant from the air before it is inhaled. To be classified as a respirator, the device must certified by NIOSH. When a respirator is available for use, there must be a written respiratory protection program and assignment of supervisory responsibility with at least the following elements in place including: (1) the facility must have procedures regarding the selection, storage, and cleaning of reusable respirators; 2) fit testing to determine whether a respiratory protective device fits a particular health-care worker; 3) fit checking that is performed before each use of the respiratory protective device by the health-care worker to check the fit; 4) medical evaluation of the health care worker to be sure the wearing of the device is not precluded; and 5) training of the users including an explanation of a description of TB hazards in their facility, why the device has been selected, an explanation of the operation, capabilities, and limitations of the respiratory protective device provided; instruction on how it should be inspected, put on, fit checked, and correctly worn, and instructions on how to know if it is malfunctioning; and 6) the effectiveness of the program should be evaluated at least yearly and whenever inspections and results of monitoring activities indicate a problem (Centers for Disease Control and Prevention, 1994).

REMOVAL FROM ISOLATION

A patient suspected of having active pulmonary or laryngeal TB must remain in isolation until determined to be noninfectious. This can occur either as a result of the medical work-up ruling out TB or the patient with active TB being placed on effective chemotherapy for an appropriate length of time, with the subsequent return of AFB smears to negative. It is recommended that a patient have at least three negative AFB sputum smears on different days before either TB is ruled out, or the patient is considered no longer infectious if the smears were previously positive. Even if the smears are negative, if the patient continues to be highly suspicious for TB, TB isolation should remain in effect.

Patients who are either AFB smear positive, or smear negative but suspected of having active TB, should be still considered to be infectious. These patients may come off isolation when they are determined to no longer be infectious. The length of time before a patient becomes noninfectious while on effective anti-TB medication varies. This decision cannot be based exclusively on a period of time but must include an evaluation of the patient's response to the medication and clinical improvement in the patient that includes reduction in coughing, absence of fever, and a progressive decrease in quantity of AFB seen on sputum smear. Some patients, particularly those with drug-resistant TB, can remain infectious for months (Centers for Disease Control and Prevention, 1994). The facility should have guidelines as to when TB isolation may be discontinued, which include the above considerations. If the culture results indicate the presence of a *Mycobacterium* other than tuberculosis, isolation may be discontinued. It is important to evaluate the patient's response to treatment to prevent patients with multidrug-resistant TB from coming off isolation at a time when they are still infectious. There should be a determination made by the Infection Control Committee as to whether a patient with known or suspected multidrug-resistant TB should ever be removed from TB isolation while in the facility because the infectious period of these patients is not known.

MONITORING AND EVALUATION OF THE TB CONTROL PROGRAM

Within a health care facility, there must be ongoing monitoring and evaluation of the TB control program to determine if nosocomial transmission of TB to staff and patients is occurring. The risk of TB in the population served by the facility should be known. Health-care workers should receive baseline tuberculin skin tests on employment which are repeated at least every 12 months to identify those who have become infected with *M. tuberculosis*. If there is a high risk of exposure to patients with active TB, the frequency of skin testing should be more frequent such as every 3 to 6 months. Those who have reactive skin tests should be evaluated for active TB and appropriate therapy begun. Data should be systematically and routinely collected on the number and percentage of skin test conversions among health-care workers and their work location (including a determination of whether the infection was nosocomial or community acquired), the number of active cases of TB among health-care workers (determination of nosocomial or community acquired), the number of TB exposures, where the exposure occurred and if it was preventable, the number of patients seen with *Mycobacterium tuberculosis*, and the incidence of MDR-TB. Analysis of these data must allow for rapid identification of problems including detection of any outbreaks, so that immediate corrective action can be taken. Guidelines must be in place for procedures to handle exposure to a patient with TB. Close contacts, defined as health care workers directly assigned to the care of the patient, should be identified. These are the individuals who are most likely to have been infected because of prolonged sharing of the air space with the patient. If there are no tuberculin skin test conversions in this group, further investigation for contacts is not necessary.

For employees identified as close contacts who have a history of a

TABLE 9.2 Education and Training of Health-Care Workers

- The basic concepts of TB transmission, pathogenesis, and diagnosis, including the difference between latent TB infection and active TB disease, the signs and symptoms of TB, and the possibility of reinfection
- The potential for occupational exposure to persons with infectious TB in the health-care facility, including the prevalence of TB in the community and facility, the ability of the facility to appropriately isolate patients with active TB, and situations with increased risk of exposure to TB.
- The principles and practices of infection control that reduce the risk of transmission of TB, including the hierarchy of TB infection control measures and the written policies and procedures of the facility. Site-specific control measures should be provided to personnel in areas that require control of TB measures in addition to the basic control program.
- The purpose of PPD testing, the significance of a positive result and the importance of participation in the skin test program.
- The principles of preventive therapy for latent TB infection. Indications, use and effectiveness including the potential adverse effects of the drugs.
- The responsibility of the health-care worker to seek medical evaluation promptly if symptoms develop that may be due to TB or if PPD test conversion occurs in order to receive appropriate evaluation and therapy and to prevent transmission of TB to patients and other health-care workers.
- The principles of drug therapy for active TB.
- The importance of notifying the facility if the health-care worker is diagnosed with active TB so appropriate contact investigation can be instituted.
- The responsibilities of the facility to maintain the confidentiality of the health-care worker, while assuring that the health-care worker with TB receives appropriate therapy and is noninfectious before returning to duty.
- The higher risk posed by TB to individuals with HIV infection or other causes of severely impaired cell-mediated immunity including (1) the more frequent and rapid development of clinical TB after infection with *M. tuberculosis* (2) the differences in the clinical presentation of disease; and (3) the high mortality rate associated with MDR-TB disease in such individuals.
- The potential development of cutaneous anergy as immune function, measured by CD4+ T-lymphocyte counts, declines.
- The facility's policy on voluntary work reassignment options for noncompromised health-care workers should be explained.
- Information on efficacy and safety of BCG vaccination

Adapted from Centers for Disease Control (1994). Guidelines for preventing the transmission of *Mycobacterium tuberculosis* in health-care facilities, 1994. *Morbidity and Mortality Weekly Report*, *43* (RR-13), 36–37.

negative tuberculin skin test more than 3 months prior to the exposure, a baseline Mantoux test performed by the intracutaneous injection of 5 tuberculin units of purified protein derivative (PPD) should be given (See Chapter 8). The test must be repeated 12 weeks after the date of the last exposure to the patient. Prior to the repeat Mantoux test, culture results on the patient should be obtained. This type of testing is discussed in Chapter 8. If the patient has an atypical *Mycobacterium* instead of *M. tuberculosis*, no exposure has occurred and no further testing is necessary. Patients determined to have been exposed to another patient with active TB should also be tested. Any employee suspected of active laryngeal or pulmonary TB must be removed from work until the medical work-up is completed and the employee is determined either not to have TB or to no longer be infectious if active TB is found. The appropriate exposure work-up must be carried out as described above.

COUNSELING AND EDUCATION OF HEALTH-CARE WORKERS

Education regarding TB should be provided for both the employees within a health-care facility and for patients diagnosed with TB. A TB education resource guide that lists educational materials, both written as well as audiovisual, is available from the American Lung Association (also see Appendix 3). Employees should receive information about TB that is appropriate to both their job responsibilities and level of understanding. This education should be updated periodically or if job assignments change so that new responsibilities with regard to TB transmission may be understood. Elements that should be included are summarized in Table 9.2.

Patients with TB should receive education about transmission of TB, importance of evaluation of their contacts for TB, treatment of TB to include medications to take and side effects of the medications, when to report problems to the physician or health care provider, and need for adherence to the treatment regimen to prevent the development of drug resistance (also see Chapters 5,6 and 7).

DISINFECTION AND STERILIZATION

Since TB is spread through the respiratory route, fomites, such as clothing, linen, food trays, walls, beds, and the like do not play a role in transmission, although transmission by bronchoscopes have been demonstrated (Centers for Disease Control and Prevention, 1994). Routine cleaning of the environment should be done first by using a detergent or disinfectant/detergent to remove any visible dirt or body fluids. The area is then disinfected with an Environmental Protection Agency (EPA)-registered chemical disinfectant such as a phenolic germicidal detergent solution (Rutala, 1990).

Instruments or devices that come into contact with sterile tissue or blood must be sterile. This includes items such as surgical instruments, implants, needles, and cardiac and urinary catheters. Equipment that comes in contact with mucous membranes or skin that is not intact should either be sterilized or receive high-level disinfection (i.e., glutaraldehyde) prior to use. This includes bronchoscopes and respiratory and anesthesia equipment. The high-level disinfection procedure will destroy ordinary vegetative bacteria, most fungal spores, tubercle bacilli, and the small nonlipid viruses. Each item that is reprocessed by disinfection or sterilization must first be thoroughly cleaned by utilizing detergent, water and mechanical friction to remove soil and organic material (Centers for Disease Control and Prevention, 1994).

After discharge of the patient who has been on TB isolation, there must be adequate time provided for the room to rid itself of airborne droplet nuclei. In the standard isolation room with six air exchanges per hour, 70 minutes are required for this to occur. This time assures a removal efficiency of 99.9%. Anyone entering the room before this time must wear a protective respiratory device.

HOME HEALTH CARE

Health-care workers visiting a patient in the home must be aware of the risks of transmission of TB in this setting. In home settings, not all the infection control measures can be in place (e.g., air handling), but the health-care workers can still have many protective precautions available to them. The air in a house or apartment of a patient with infectious pulmonary or laryngeal TB must be assumed to contain infectious droplet nuclei. Therefore, prior to entering, the health-care worker must put on a properly fitted respiratory protective device and remove it after leaving. Health-care workers who are using cough inducing procedures, such as inducing sputum for AFB smear or culture should also wear a respiratory protective device, and be sure the area is well ventilated and away from other household members. Once the patient is determined to be noninfectious this is no longer necessary (Centers for Disease Control and Prevention, 1994).

There needs to be ongoing evaluation of the patient for adherence to treatment as long as home visits continue. Whenever there is a concern about nonadherence to anti-TB medication, the health-care worker may need to resume the use of the respiratory protective device until the patient is again determined to be noninfectious. Directly observed therapy (DOT) may be instituted.

Education of the patient should include information regarding the need for adherence to treatment, both for taking the anti-TB medications and attending the medical appointments. The patient should cover his or her mouth and nose with a tissue when coughing or sneezing. All contacts should be referred to the local health department for tuberculin skin and other testing for tuberculous infection and/or tuberculosis and started on appropriate therapy if needed.

Patients who require transportation by a health-care worker should wear a surgical mask if infectious. If unable to do this, then the health care worker should wear a respiratory protective device. Masks are used by TB patients to prevent droplet nuclei explusion into the air. Particulate respirators are used to filter air before inhalation and protect the health care worker (CDC 1994). An additional protection is to keep the windows open to provide an exchange of air. The heater or air-conditioning unit should not be placed on recirculation of air in the transport vehicle but should bring in fresh air.

ROLE OF THE HEALTH-CARE WORKER

The effectiveness of an infection control program to prevent the nosocomial transmission of *Mycobacterium tuberculosis* depends on the dedication of the employees to follow established TB control policies and procedures. There is always a risk of exposure to patients with active pulmonary or laryngeal TB. The key to minimizing this risk is for the health care worker to maintain a high index of suspicion, rapid identification of TB cases, prompt placement of these patients on TB isolation, and close adherence to other infection control measures. Only through constant vigilance can health-care workers prevent nosocomial transmission of *Mycobacterium tuberculosis*.

REFERENCES

Centers for Disease Control. (1989). Prevention and control of tuberculosis in correctional institutions: Recommendations of the Advisory Committee for the Elimination of Tuberculosis. *Morbidity and Mortality Weekly Report, 38*, 313–320, 325.
Centers for Disease Control. (1990a). Guidelines for preventing the transmission of tuberculosis in health-care settings, with special focus on HIV-related issues. *Morbidity and Mortality Weekly Report, 39*, (RR–17).
Centers for Disease Control. (1990b). Prevention and control of tuberculosis in facilities providing long-term care to the elderly. *Morbidity and Mortality Weekly Report, 39*, (RR–10).
Centers for Disease Control. (1991) Nosocomial transmission of multidrug-

resistant tuberculosis among HIV-infected persons-Florida and New York, 1988–1991. *Morbidity and Mortality Weekly Report, 40,* 585–591.

Centers for Disease Control. (1994). Guidelines for preventing the transmission of *Mycobacterium tuberculosis* in health-care facilities, 1994. *Morbidity and Mortality Weekly Report, 43* (RR-13), 1–133.

Fraser, V.J., Johnson, K., Primack, J., Jones, M., Medoff, G., & Dunagan, W. C. (1993). Evaluation of rooms with negative pressure ventilation used for respiratory isolation in seven midwestern hospitals. *Infection Control and Hospital Epidemiology, 14,* 623–628.

Health Resources and Services Administration. (1984). *Guidelines for construction and equipment of hospital and medical facilities.* (PHS Publication no.(HRSA)84–14500). Rockville, MD: US Department of Health & Human Services, Public Health Services.

Nardell, E.A. (1993). Environmental control of tuberculosis. *Medical Clinics of North America, 77(6),* 1315–1334.

National Institute for Occupational Safety and Health. (1981). *Occupational Respiratory Protection (593).* (publication no.593). Cincinnati, OH: US Department of Health and Human Services, Public Health Service, Centers for Disease Control, National Institute for Occupational Safety and Health.

Nicas, M., Sprinson, J. E., Royce, S. E., Harrison, R. J., & Macher, J. M. (1993). Isolation rooms for tuberculosis control. *Infection Control and Hospital Epidemiology, 14,* 619–622.

Riley, R. L. (1993). Transmission and environmental control of tuberculosis. *Lung Biology in Health and Disease, 66,* 123–136.

Riley, R. L., Mills, C. C., O'Grady, F., Sultan, L. U., Wittstadt, F., Shivpuri, D. N. (1962). Infectiousness of air from a tuberculosis ward. *American Review of Respiratory Disease, 85,* 511–525.

Rutala, W. A. (1990). APIC guideline for selection and use of disinfectants. *American Journal of Infection Control, 18,* 99–117.

Ultraviolet faces revival to fight TB. *The New York Times,* January 4, 1994, B1.

U.S. Department of Health and Human Resources. NIOSH recommended guidelines for personal respiratory protection of working in health care facilities potentially exposed to tuberculosis. Atlanta: Author, 1994.

10

COMMUNITY-BASED STRATEGIES FOR TUBERCULOSIS CONTROL

Janice A. Boutotte and Sue Etkind

Tuberculosis (TB) control activities had their origin in the early 1900s in the public health arena through the efforts of local community health nurses in urban cities. These nurses were charged with the home-based care of persons afflicted with TB prior to the advent of medications for tuberculosis. As the role of public health became more formalized, TB outpatient medical care expanded and became a major activity for physicians, nurses, and others charged with "protecting the public's health" (Bates, 1992).

Current trends in the delivery of health care support a shift to community-based care. Given the problems with patient adherence to prescribed TB treatment, ensuring that patients complete the prescribed therapeutic regimen with the long-term administration of medications often requires a comprehensive approach beyond that of the traditional TB clinic. Therefore, to control TB, innovative strategies for caring for clients in the community must be designed and developed. This chapter focuses on the both the traditional and innovative tuberculosis control activities provided by public health departments. Traditional activities include case finding, contact investigation, and nursing case management; innovative strategies and models of care include the use of incentives and enablers to promote adherence to therapy, public-private partnerships, and community-based educational campaigns.

PUBLIC HEALTH DEPARTMENT TUBERCULOSIS CONTROL ACTIVITIES

The public health department is the usual state agency that has the delegated legal responsibility for control of infectious diseases. The precise laws and regulations governing these agencies vary from state to state, but the overall mandate of the protection of the public health remains constant (Etkind, 1993a). In a 50-state survey of TB statutes, Gostin (1993) reported that all states "exercised their police powers to control the spread of communicable diseases, including TB (Gostin, 1993, p. 255). These included medical examination, treatment, emergency detention, commitment to state facilities, isolation, and quarantine with the imposition of criminal penalties for "knowing transmission" of TB (Gostin, 1993). Some of these may be out of date or inadequate, and one of the objectives of the National Action Plan to Combat Multidrug-resistant TB (See Appendix 2) is to develop recommendations regarding TB control (Centers for Disease Control, 1992b). TB control activities of the public health department include surveillance, case finding, TB case registries, and contact tracing. These are discussed below.

Surveillance

Surveillance, the systematic collection of data, is a function traditionally carried out by health departments and allows the recognition of trends in a disease as well as providing morbidity and mortality information (Centers for Disease Control, 1992b). Surveillance has typically been done passively by receiving reports from hospitals, clinics, and other health care providers of a confirmed or suspected case of TB and begins when the responsible health care provider (usually the physician) reports the case. Prompt reporting allows not only the ensurance of adequate TB care for the individual with TB but also allows for the investigation of contacts and the detection of other cases as discussed later in this chapter (Etkind, 1993a). Public health departments need to be able to identify groups of persons in the community among whom tuberculosis is occurring because of the risk of possible transmission of infection. This identification may require the collection and analysis of data not always included on agency case reports, such as institutional residence, occupation, socioeconomic status indicators, alcohol and other substance abuse, and HIV antibody status (Centers for Disease Control, 1989). In July 1993, the CDC distributed a new computer software package (SUR-VS-TB) to state and local health departments. This package is used to transfer records to CDC after completing the Report of a Verified Case of TB (RVCT) form. Additional information collected now includes occupation, history of substance abuse, HIV testing results, homelessness, residence in a correctional or long-term-care facility, initial therapy, type of health-care provider, sputum culture conversion, and use of directly observed therapy (DOT) (Centers for Disease Control and Prevention, 1994a). Community assessment data concerning the prevalence of TB in a specific area, the at-risk groups affected in the community, and drug resistance rates can then be available to local health care providers to assist them in making decisions relative to diagnosis, treatment, and follow-up (Etkind, 1993a).

Case Finding

Case finding is the identification of those infected with *M. tuberculosis* in order to provide appropriate therapy and quickly interrupt transmission (Rieder, 1993). Traditional methods of case finding include 1) receiving reports of cases from sources such as providers and screening programs in order to target persons at risk for tuberculous infection and 2) conducting contact investigations. Area health care providers should be encouraged to report a suspected case as early as possible and not wait for confirmatory reports, because this may result in continued transmission, a delay in the screening of contacts of the case, and possibly the development of drug-resistant disease if the person with TB is nonadherent to treatment or lost to follow-up. The CDC recommend that cases should be reported to the health department within 3 days (Centers for Disease Control, 1989). New computer software for surveillance should assist in this process (Centers for Disease Control and Prevention, 1994a). Nurses working within health departments can help implement strategies to improve reporting by using new technological methods to make the process easier, such as 24-hour telephone reporting with the use of answering machines, electronic transfer of reports via computers (especially from facilities that report cases frequently), and mechanisms to ensure notification of positive bacteriology and drug sensitivity reports from laboratories, such as electronic linkages or laboratory reporting laws.

Today, some health departments are also utilizing more active methods of surveillance for case finding, such as validation studies to evaluate the completeness of reporting of cases through periodic matching of TB and acquired immunodeficiency syndrome (AIDS) case registries, review of laboratory and pharmacy reports, death registry and hospital discharge tapes, and periodic record audits. Although many of these activities may be done by nonprofessional staff, nurses should be involved in designing and implementing the systems to verify that the appropriate information is obtained and to ensure client confidentiality.

Tuberculosis Case Registries

Health departments have also traditionally maintained TB case registries. These registries keep information on all actual and suspected cases of TB. The registries were designed initially for case management purposes and were usually maintained as paper records. Recent advances in epidemiology, enhanced computer capacities, and an increased emphasis on the importance of surveillance in targeting TB control activities have contributed to a change in the case registry concept. Although surveillance capacities vary depending on local resources, registry data may include patient demographic data, clinical information pertaining to the disease presentation, and the level of infectiousness, treatment regimens, clinical progress, recommendations, and health-care follow-up (Etkind, 1993a).

In some areas, the case registry concept has been expanded to include registries of contacts to cases, persons on preventive therapy, registries of persons with both tuberculosis and AIDS, and registries of specific populations with tuberculosis, such as homeless persons, children, persons in drug treatment centers, institutionalized persons (especially correctional inmates), and health care-workers.

CONTACT INVESTIGATION

Risk identification, or "contact investigation or tracing" as it is more commonly called, identifies those persons who are at greatest risk of having been infected with TB by the presenting or index case and who are at high risk for progression to disease. It is estimated that the average number of contacts identified for each case of TB in the United States is nine. Successful contact tracing requires skills in patient assessment, interviewing, counseling, and evaluation (Etkind, 1993b). It has traditionally been carried out by public health nurses, but is also done in hospitals and other institutions when a suspect case of TB is identified in a patient or health care worker in conjunction with the health department to ensure that community contacts are also screened.

Contact investigation is initiated as soon as a confirmed or suspected case of TB is identified and should begin within 3 days by a person trained in contact interviewing (Centers for Disease Control, 1989). The nurse begins the epidemiological process by collecting all currently available information about the presenting case in a systematic fashion during the nursing assessment. After this information is collected, the nurse can then complete the process by interviewing the case and/or family contacts. This can be done in the hospital or clinic, in the client's home, or other location convenient for the client and conducive to establishing trust and rapport. A visit to the contact's place of employment may also be necessary. The ability to conduct an interview to obtain client and contact information will determine the success or failure of the investigation (American Thoracic Society, 1992; Etkind, 1993b). Use of an interpreter may be necessary when interviewing some clients. From the information, a list of contacts with whom the suspect or case has had contact should be generated along with information on how to locate them.

When conducting the contact investigation, it is important to set limits and establish priorities. Without a systematic approach to the process, persons who are not at demonstrated risk of tuberculous infection or tuberculosis may be screened. Prior to the actual field investigation the contact tracing should be focused on identifying those at highest risk by assessing the risk of TB transmission to identified contacts (American Thoracic Society, 1992; Etkind, 1993b). Factors influencing this include patient, environmental, and contact characteristics along with time considerations (the duration and frequency of exposure) (American Thoracic Society, 1992).

The nurse should first determine the infectiousness of the presenting case by considering individual clinical factors. Usually, a person can only be considered to be infectious if the site of disease is pulmonary or in the upper respiratory system. If the person has a positive sputum smear or culture, lung cavitation, history of a frequent productive cough for several weeks or more, thin, watery secretions, has been on inadequate anti-TB therapy, hemoptysis, or is hoarse, or has undergone cough-inducing procedures such as aerosolized pentamidine treatment, then the likelihood of disease transmission is high and the need for rapid contact tracing is clear (American Thoracic Society, 1992).

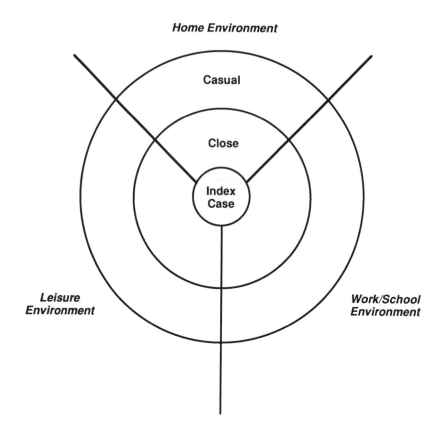

FIGURE 10.1 Contact tracing using the concentric circle method.

Source: Iseman, M. D. (1979). Containment of tuberculosis. *Chest, 76,* (suppl. 6), 804. ´

Next, the nurse should establish the duration and frequency of exposure, e.g., how long the contacts were potentially exposed to the case
during the infectious stage. The onset of symptoms, particularly coughing, should be used to gauge the approximate time from which contacts
were exposed until the exposure has ended or the source case became
noninfectious. In the absence of coughing, some consider the beginning
of the infectious period as 3 months before the date of the first abnormal
chest radiograph, positive sputum smear or culture or histologic study.

When infectiousness is considered to end is not entirely clear (Noble, 1981). Previous estimates that infectiousness ends after 2 weeks of therapy have not been substantiated by data; some patients may remain infectious for several weeks or months depending upon the adequacy of their treatment and the drug-susceptibility or resistance of the strain of *M. tuberculosis*. Therefore, the CDC recommend that infectiousness be evaluated on a case-by-case basis. In general, a person on adequate chemotherapy with significant clinical and bacteriologic response to therapy is no longer infectious; however, the patient should be considered so until three consecutive sputum smears are negative and/or there is clinical improvement if sputum smears were not obtained (Centers for Disease Control and Prevention, 1994b).

After determining the level of potential infectivity of the case and the time frame during which possible exposures may have occurred, the investigating nurse should establish the place (or places) where contacts may have been exposed, keeping in mind that the risk of transmission is greatest for contacts who have spent the most time in close contact (particularly sharing the same indoor environment) with the case; thus, household contacts are at highest risk. Other potential places of transmission are shelters, the workplace, schools, and health care and other institutions. In addition to deciding the possible locations of exposure, the nurse should obtain additional information about the environmental factors of the sites, such as 1) ventilation; 2) degree and direction of airflow; 3) volume of air common to the source patient and contact (the size off the rooms); 4) the presence or absence of ultraviolet lighting; 5) the presence or absence of high efficency particulate air (HEPA) filters; and 6) the number of people sharing the same space (American Thoracic Society, 1992).

After considering the transmission risk, contact tracing priorities using the concentric-circle approach should be established (see Figure 10.1), identifying contacts at home, work, school, and leisure settings (Iseman, 1979). Persons from each of these settings with the highest risk of infection (exposure to a potentially highly infectious case for extended periods of time in the same place, usually household contacts) are in the concentric circle immediately next to the index case. Those in this first or inner circle should be offered tuberculin skin testing and be referred for medical evaluation. If the percentage of contacts testing positive is greater than would be expected in the general population, then the next circle of contacts should be screened, that is, those who have frequently breathed the same indoor air as the case, but not as often as the close contacts. The next circle includes frequent visitors, relatives, and co-workers. The circle of contacts being tested should widen as long as the infection rate in the contacts being tested remains above the expected

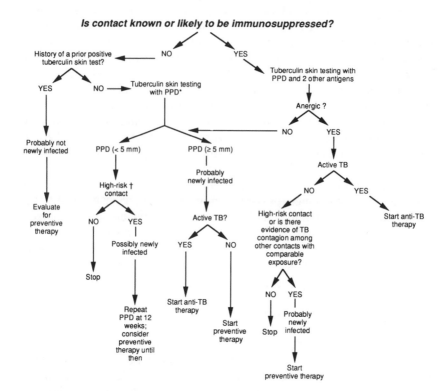

FIGURE 10.2 Preventive therapy decision making for contracts of infectious tuberculosis cases.

Sources: Centers for Disease Control and Prevention (1992a). Management of persons exposed to multidrug-resistant tuberculosis. *Morbidity and Mortality Weekly Report, 41,* (No. RR-11), p. 63.

general population rate. The investigation should stop when a circle of contacts is found who have no more infection than is expected in the community. Contacts who test negative for the initial tuberculin skin test should be retested again in 3 months, unless tuberculosis has been ruled out in the suspect case. If the exposure continues to the index case, contacts should be retested every 3 months until exposure has ended.

Contact is broken when the index case is no longer infectious or the contact is physically removed from exposure. Contacts identified should have a complete diagnostic evaluation, and those with symptoms of TB should be placed on an appropriate treatment regimen (Centers for Disease Control, 1992a). Those with no evidence of disease should be considered for preventive therapy. Those who have a tuberculin reaction of 5 mm or more should have a chest radiograph and if no clinical disease is found should be considered for preventive therapy. Those who have a tuberculin reaction of less than 5 mm should receive a chest radiograph and be considered for preventive therapy, even though the tuberculin skin test is not positive and clinical disease is not evident under the following conditions: 1) there is a high probability of infection, 2) the contact is a child or adolescent, has HIV-infection or is otherwise immunosuppressed; or 3) has exposure similar to contacts of the index case who have already become infected (American Thoracic Society, 1992). A flow chart for preventive therapy decision making is shown in Figure 10.2.

CASE MANAGEMENT—A MULTIDISCIPLINARY-MULTIFACTORIAL APPROACH

Patient adherence to prescribed tuberculosis treatment is the major obstacle facing health care providers today (Sumartojo, 1993; also see Chapter 7). Public health departments must now provide an array of services based on an assessment of what is needed to get clients to complete therapy. These services may simply be providing education, information, and consultative support to the health-care provider who has the resources to provide case management and contact investigations or, more often, the actual provision of resources to assist in the management of the case. These resources may need to be multidisciplinary and employ a variety of individualized approaches to assist patients in completing therapy (Etkind, 1993a).

An effective approach to help patients complete TB treatment is the use of a case management model. According to Bower (1992), "The fundamental focus of case management is to integrate, coordinate, and advocate for individuals, families, and groups requiring extensive services . . . assuring that clients receive appropriate, individualized, and cost-effective care within a system of services" (p. 3).

The CDC have recommended that for each new case of TB, a specific health department employee be assigned the responsibility and accountability for ensuring that 1) the client receives education about TB and its treatment; 2) the client completes an appropriate course of therapy;

and 3) contacts are identified and examined (Centers for Disease Control, 1989). These are all essential components of case management. When the health department receives a report of a case of confirmed or suspected active tuberculosis, it should be immediately assigned to a single public health nurse who will be responsible for delivering or coordinating all of the client's care until the client is discharged from the system.

Nursing Case Management

Community service coordination was a forerunner of case management in the early 1900s and has always been a focus of public health nursing (Grau, 1984). Nurses are particularly suited to provide case management for clients with multiple health problems requiring long-term follow-up because of their substantial clinical knowledge, skills, and judgement (Mundinger, 1984). Nurses assist clients, facilitating their adaptation to potential or actual effects of health disruptions. They practice with extensive knowledge of the multifaceted issues presented by clients and their families, including the physical and psychosocial dimensions (Bower, 1992). As a process, case management expands on the components of the nursing process: assessment, goal/outcome development, planning, intervention, monitoring, and evaluation. Utilization of the nursing case management model in the follow-up of tuberculosis clients provides a framework within which to deliver quality nursing care and effect positive outcomes. The following sections describe some specific strategies and examples of the use of this model in TB control.

Nursing Assessment. Case management requires the development of relationships among the nurse case manager, client, family members, and other service providers. Trust and support are built through effective communication techniques that foster these relationships (Bower, 1992). This is particularly important in TB control because many of the clients are from countries or cultures differing from those of the care provider where English may not be well-understood or spoken, or have additional problems such as homelessness, substance use dependency, or other medical problems. The nurse should perform a nursing assessment takes into account the patient's personal and psychosocial needs, factors may affect adherence to prescribed treatment, access to appropriate health care, and barriers to care, such as cultural or linguistic differences. After the data are collected, analyzed, and synthesized, the nurse should formulate nursing diagnoses and other interdisciplinary problem statements.

The nurse should obtain a history of the client, first collecting as much information as possible before talking to the client. Data can be obtained through review of the medical records (hospital, clinic, or other records, including laboratory reports) and from the health care provider or other reporting source. It is important to know the clinical history and results of tests to assist in determining the level of infectiousness of the patient. Information obtained should include the disease site, dates, sources and bacteriological results for acid-fast bacilli (AFB) smears and cultures, chest radiograph results, including the extent of disease and whether it is cavitary or noncavitary, skin test results, clinical signs and symptoms (including frequency and characteristics of any productive, nonproductive, cough, hemoptysis), and duration of illness. The nurse should contact the client's physician to find out if instructions were given regarding any activity restrictions, such as length of time to be absent from work, and the prescribed antituberculosis drug regimen, including dosages and date initiated. The nurse should also inquire if the physician has tested any of the client's contacts and if interpretive services will be needed to communicate with the client.

The nurse should then contact the client to schedule a convenient time to make a home visit to interview the client and family. When interviewing the client, it is important to try to elicit information that will help determine the person's potential risk for nonadherence (See Chapter 7), for example, a history of substance abuse or enrollment in treatment programs (alcohol, injecting drugs, crack, and cocaine), homelessness, history of incarceration, different cultural perceptions of health and illness (particularly TB), and the patient's previous history of showing up for health care appointments and following prescribed treatments. A history of previous antituberculosis treatment, for either preventive therapy or active disease, can provide an indication not only of potential nonadherence but also of possible drug resistance (see Chapter 5). The assessment should also include looking for any medical risk factors that, if present, might affect the course of disease, such as HIV infection, cancer, immunosuppressive therapy (including corticosteroid use), and diabetes. Since HIV coinfection is a growing problem, the nurse should do an HIV risk assessment and, if any risks are present, the nurse should encourage the person to seek HIV counseling and testing. If a tuberculin skin test has not been done already, skin testing using the Mantoux technique should be arranged.

Plan of Care. The next phase of case management is the development of an individualized care plan with client participation. Together, the nurse and client should set mutually agreed-upon goals with measurable objectives, determine action steps toward goal achievement, and select essential resources and services through collaboration among health care professionals, the client, and the family (Bower, 1992).

The nursing care plan for clients with TB should include interventions to ensure the following outcomes: 1) completion of an effective, uninterrupted course of therapy, including following current treatment recommendations that include drugs to which the organisms are susceptible (American Thoracic Society, 1994. Centers for Disease Control and Prevention, 1993; Wolinsky, 1993); 2) the shortest therapy course possible to enhance adherence to the prescribed regimen, including taking medications as prescribed; and 3) regular monitoring for side effects of medications and response to therapy (Boutotte, 1993).

Implementation. The implementation phase provides for the delivery of care by linking the client with appropriate service providers. In some models of case management, the nurse is both a provider of direct nursing care and the coordinator of services or is the latter only with the direct care provided by others (Bower, 1992). In TB control, community outreach workers are often utilized to provide some of the direct care, particularly to diverse populations. These outreach workers should work under the supervision of a nurse, who will be responsible for supervising the outreach workers, delegating assignments, coordinating the client's care, assessing outcomes, and making other appropriate community referrals (American Nurses Association, 1993; Boskovich, 1994).

Evaluation. This phase of the process includes ongoing monitoring and assessment of the client's progress. The nurse should maintain contact with the client, the client's support systems, and direct service providers in order to continually evaluate the client's responses to interventions and progress toward the preestablished goals. As new information is obtained, the nursing diagnoses and goals may need to be modified. Ongoing care coordination is necessary until the desired outcomes are achieved. Undesired outcomes must also be evaluated.

In TB control, the nurse evaluates the client's response to therapy by obtaining follow-up samples of sputum weekly until the sputum cultures are negative. Persistent positive sputum cultures (particularly after 3 months of therapy) are a definitive sign of treatment failure or relapse, and the persistence or reappearance of organisms in the smear should create a high index of suspicion for the presence of drug-resistance or nonadherence to therapy (Centers for Disease Control and Prevention, 1993). In addition, at each client encounter, the nurse should monitor the client for any signs of adverse drug reactions through interviews and periodic liver function tests and for adherence to therapy through interviews, pill counts, and urine tests (Boutotte, 1993; also see Chapter 5).

The Use of Community Outreach Workers

Most states and large cities have some outreach capacity within the TB program. These workers represent the social or cultural background of the client and are often able to establish a relationship with the client that is much stronger than that of the traditional medical establishment. Successful outreach programs often employ workers from the same ethnic and/or cultural background, workers who are recovered addicts or formerly homeless, persons from the same neighborhood or housing project, or respected church or community members.

The education and training of the outreach worker is critical and should be done by a professional nurse who maintains the accountability for the care of the client being carried out by the outreach worker. The tasks and functions of the outreach worker need to be clearly delineated from those of the nurse, including specific instructions regarding what information to report back to the nurse. Examples of tasks that can be delegated to outreach workers include: following up on clients who fail to keep scheduled appointments, collecting sputum specimens, doing pill counts, performing directly observed therapy (DOT), reinforcing the patient teaching on TB done by the nurse or other health-care provider, providing interpreter services, and administering and/or reading tuberculin skin tests (after specialized training).

The Use of Directly Observed Therapy

Directly observed therapy (DOT) is one method of ensuring the client's adherence to treatment by requiring that a health care provider or other designated person observe the client ingest the TB medication(s). DOT can be administered daily or 2 to 3 times weekly. The client and nurse should agree on a method that ensures the best possible DOT routine and maintains confidentiality. It has been recently recommended that DOT be considered for all patients because it is difficult to predict which patients will adhere to a prescribed treatment regimen (Centers for Disease Control and Prevention, 1993).

Although DOT is an effective strategy that is being recommended by CDC and others (American Thoracic Society, 1994; Centers for Disease Control and Prevention, 1993; Iseman, Cohn, & Sbarbaro, 1993), it is a more restrictive measure than self-administered therapy and more re-

**TABLE 10.1 A Progressive, Stepwise, Case-Management Approach
To Tuberculosis Treatment**

Least Restrictive	1.	Self administered, daily, short-course therapy with monthly clinic visits.
	2.	Directly observed therapy (DOT), twice or thrice weekly, fully supervised in clinic, home or alternative site.
	3.	Voluntary long-term hospitalization in a specialized tuberculosis treatment unit.
Most Restrictive	4.	Compulsory, court-ordered, long-term hospitalization in a secure tuberculosis treatment unit

Source: Nardell, E. A. (1993). Beyond four drugs, *American Review of Respiratory Disease, 148*, p. 4.

source intensive. Approaches to TB treatment are shown in Table 10.1. One of the primary goals of the nursing assessment is to determine if DOT will be necessary based on the client's risk factors for nonadherence, acuity level of disease (infectiousness, risk of MDR-TB, etc.), other relevant social factors, such as cultural or ethnic barriers, and available resources. If the assessment suggests a potential for nonadherence, DOT should be implemented at the start of therapy. It must be kept in mind that nonadherence may be difficult to predict (see Chapter 7). Frequently, health care providers wait until the client has not completed the treatment as prescribed (sometimes several times) before initiating DOT; in these circumstances, DOT may be viewed by the client as a punitive measure and result in increased resistance. If DOT is implemented at the beginning of therapy as the standard of care for that client, it is usually received more favorably and has the desired outcome of completion of therapy.

Effective use of DOT may require an outreach worker to go into the community to locate a client and observe the ingestion of each dose of medication. However, DOT can be done in TB or AIDS clinics, community health centers, migrant clinics, homeless shelters, prisons or jails, nursing homes, schools, drug treatment centers, or occupational sites. In some situations, a responsible person other than a health-care worker may administer DOT, such as correctional facility personnel, staff of community-based organizations (CBO), teachers, reliable volunteers, social workers, drug treatment center staff, clergy, or other community leaders (Centers for Disease Control and Prevention, 1993). These arrangements require careful supervision by the nurse and ongoing coordination of services. DOT is not foolproof; the astute client may avoid adhering to a medication regimen even under DOT (See Chapter 7).

Incentives and Enablers

Another strategy that can be used to encourage clients to complete therapy is the use of incentives and/or enablers. Incentives are defined as "motivators," something that motivates a client to take the medication and keep clinic appointments, such as food or coffee at the clinic; food coupons; individualized articles, such as socks for the homeless; or cash (Etkind, 1993b; Pozsik, 1993). Enablers is a term used to describe anything that assists (enables) the client to more readily complete therapy or access services, such as transportation, bus and transit tokens, child care, free medications, and evening clinic hours (Pozsik, 1993). The use of incentives is discussed in greater detail in Chapter 7.

EDUCATIONAL ACTIVITIES

Public health nurses can play a significant role in providing "expert" consultation to practitioners caring for TB patients. Public health nurses are aware of local rates of TB disease and infection in specific high-risk populations. They also have many opportunities to consult with physicians on an individual client basis during the long course of treatment. Thus they play an essential role in professional education.

Client education should be integrated into all aspects of TB control and reinforced at every encounter. In recent years there have been many educational tools developed by both the CDC and various state and local programs. A summary of many of these materials can be found in the *Tuberculosis Education Resource Guide* (American Lung Association, 1993) and the Appendix 3. Many of these materials are also available in various languages. An effective client education tool is the use of videotapes, which can be shown while clients are waiting at the clinic for their appointments.

Clients may also be given handouts to take home and read, help them process more information than they would otherwise remember. When selecting educational materials for the client, consideration should be given to those that target particular high-risk groups and contain specific messages, as well as those with more general information. The materials should be at an appropriate reading level and in a language the client can read. Nurses can also be involved in the development of new materials, targeted to specific groups or for particular projects. If materials need to be translated into other languages, they should be back translated to ensure the information is translated accurately and conveys the meaning that the health-care provider intended.

MODEL PROJECTS/PUBLIC-PRIVATE PARTNERSHIPS

Some states and large cities report declining tuberculosis case rates, despite increases in cases elsewhere in the United States. Programs in these areas have utilized a variety of measures to achieve their success and target the needs of specific local population groups, using individualized treatment approaches. A few examples of model programs using innovative strategies are described in the remainder of this section.

Massachusetts Case Management Model

Massachusetts uses a nursing case management approach involving a statewide network of clinics, public health nurses, physicians, outreach workers, and other support staff. Whether an individual elects to receive treatment through one of the clinics or from a private provider, each active case of tuberculosis is assigned to one state or local health department nurse, depending on local resources. The nurse is responsible for seeing that the client completes a satisfactory course of therapy, applying whatever measures are necessary to succeed, on an individualized basis. Self-administered, daily therapy predominates statewide, but fully supervised, twice-weekly therapy is done when necessary. The premise is to use the least restrictive, but most effective, method of treatment delivery optimal for that client. Services are delivered in a culturally and linguistically appropriate manner through the use of bicultural/bilingual nurses, outreach workers, and other clinic staff. After several years of an increase in TB cases, the cases are now declining in Massachusetts led by decreases in Boston.

Mississippi Tuberculosis Program

In 1984, the state of Mississippi had 380 active TB cases with a case rate of 16.0 per 100,000 persons and was ranked fourth among the states. As a means of addressing the TB morbidity problem, the State TB Program implemented a policy of universal DOT. By 1992, the case rate had decreased to 10.8/100,000. However, other interventions have also been used in Mississippi since the onset of the DOT program, including a public health nurse-managed system, the adoption of a four-drug regimen, an intensive public relations and educational campaign, prioritization of tuberculosis patient services, decreased or eliminated waiting time for patients at clinics, an expanded incentive program to assist with transportation costs, increased outreach, and the use of restrictive measures when all else fails.

Boston Homeless Incentive Project

This project is described in detail in Chapter 12. Briefly, tuberculosis in Boston's homeless has been a particular problem since 1984, when an outbreak of drug-resistant disease occurred. Although over 90% of the homeless cases completed an adequate course of therapy, cases in the homeless continued to occur. In 1990, with private funding, an incentive program to deliver preventive therapy was initiated. Homeless persons who were candidates for therapy and agreed to participate were offered a small incentive equivalent to $6 a week to adhere to a course of directly observed preventive therapy. Clients were given food vouchers for local restaurants or cash, which could either be taken weekly or banked until the end of treatment. Preliminary results of the data appear encouraging, with the number of tuberculosis cases in the homeless decreasing during the past 2 years and the number of drug-resistant cases becoming the lowest it has been in 8 years.

Prevention and Education Models/Public-Private Partnerships

As tuberculosis puts on a ''new face,'' there have been efforts to expand TB activities beyond the public health arena and into other community services, such as community based organizations (CBOs) and other public-private partnerships. The development of these partnerships is partly based on the fact that other groups are better able to reach some of the high-risk populations and gain their trust, particularly since it is often unrealistic to expect these clients to attend a TB clinic, no matter how well it is structured to meet the clients' needs. Some of these other organizations are community health centers, substance abuse treatment programs, and other types of agencies, such as sexually transmitted disease clinics and HIV counseling and testing centers, homeless shelters, prisons and jails, and CBOs.

A very effective method of delivering educational messages is through the use of peer educators. One model of a peer education program, developed through a public-private venture in Boston, Massachusetts, is with a CBO, the Action for Boston Community Development. This CBO has recruited and trained community workers as peer educators from seven inner city housing developments. These educators are used to provide individual and group TB and HIV informational sessions through a variety of mechanisms to ensure that high-risk individuals are screened for both diseases where appropriate and evaluated medically. Workers follow any client placed on TB preventive therapy for the duration of treatment. Project directors have established linkages with both the state and city TB control programs and the local neighborhood health centers to provide comprehensive services to these residents, who might not otherwise access services. Nurses are involved in the training of the peer educators and the project has a part-time nurse consultant to assist with the case management of clients receiving preventive therapy.

Another successful model of education and prevention is the TB/HIV Prevention Project. This project is funded by the CDC in several states to provide education, screening, and the delivery of preventive therapy to clients in three types of sites: methadone maintenance treatment centers, correctional facilities, and sexually transmitted disease clinics. At the methadone treatment sites, clients entering treatment are screened for TB, referred to TB clinics for evaluation when indicated, and then receive directly observed preventive therapy onsite. Data are collected on all clients at the enrolled sites and sent to the CDC on a quarterly basis. Nurses are involved in many of these projects as program coordinators, providing client education, administering medication, and/or overseeing the data collection and analysis.

These are examples of creative strategies that can be used by nurses and other providers to assist clients in completing an adequate course of therapy for either prevention or disease.

SUMMARY

Public health departments have a crucial role to play in TB control efforts. They will continue to play such a role as community health care is strengthened, and their legal mandate to protect the public health is continued. Contact investigation is a major effort for health departments that can prevent the spread of TB. Case managment is another effort, whereby one nurse is responsible for a designated TB case to ensure completion of successful therapy. In urban areas, it has been said that the rise in TB is "not due only to HIV or homeless problems usually cited by the media, but it reflects the total failure of a public health system, even in the face of previous experience and warnings" (Reichman, 1991, p. 741). Support of public health department TB control efforts, including necessary funding for nurses, services, and programs, are necessary to strengthen the successful effort to control TB in the United States.

REFERENCES

American Lung Association. (1993). *Tuberculosis Education Resource Guide.* New York: Author.

American Nurses Association. (1993). Position statement on tuberculosis and public health nursing. Washington, DC: Author.

American Thoracic Society (1992). Control of tuberculosis in the United States. *American Review of Respiratory Disease, 146,* 1623–1633.

American Thoracic Society. (1994). Treatment of tuberculosis and tuberculosis infection in adults and children. *American Journal of Respiratory and Critical Care Medicine, 149,* 1359–1374.

Bates. B. (1992). *Bargaining for life: A social history of tuberculosis 1876–1938.* Philadelphia: University of Pennsylvania Press.

Boskovich, S. J. (1994). New concepts in nursing management of the TB patient: A community training program. *Journal of Community Health Nursing, 11(1),* 45–49.

Boutotte, J. (1993, May). T.B., the second time around . . . and how you can help to control it. *Nursing 93. 23*(5),42–50.

Bower, K. (1992). *Case management by nurses* (rev.). Kansas City, MO: American Nurses Publishing.

Centers for Disease Control. (1989). A strategic plan for the elimination of tuberculosis in the United States. *Morbidity and Mortality Weekly Report, 38,* (No. S–3), 1–25).

Centers for Disease Control adnPrevention (1992a). Management of persons exposed to multidrug-resistant tuberculosis. *Morbidity and Mortality Weekly Report, 41,* (No. RR–11), 61–71.

Centers for Disease Control (1992b). National action plan to combat multidrug-resistant tuberculosis. *Morbidity and Mortality Weekly Report, 41(RR–11),* 1–48.

Centers for Disease Control and Prevention (1993). Initial therapy for tuberculosis in the era of multidrug resistance. *Morbidity and Mortality Weekly Report, 42 (No.RR–7),* 1–8.

Centers for Disease Control. (1994b). Guidelines for preventing the transmission of *Mycobacterium tuberculosis* in health-care facilities, 1994. *Morbidity and Mortality Weekly Report, 43* (RR–13), 1–133.

Centers for Disease Control and Prevention (1994a). Expanded tuberculosis surveillance and tuberculosis morbidity—United States, 1993. *Morbidity and Mortality Weekly Report, 43,* 361–366.

Etkind, S. C. (1993a). The role of the public health department in tuberculosis. *Medical Clinics of North America, 77(6)*, 1303–1314.

Etkind, S. (1993b). Contact tracing in tuberculosis. *Lung Biology in Health and Disease, 66*, 275–288.

Gostin, L. O. (1993). Controlling the resurgent tuberculosis epidemic. *Journal of the American Medical Association, 269,* 255–261.

Grau, L. (1984). Case management and the nurse. *Geriatric Nursing 5*, 372–375.

Iseman, M.D. (1979). Containment of tuberculosis. *Chest, 76,* (suppl. 6),801–804.

Iseman, M. D., Cohn, D. L., & Sbarbaro, J. A. (1993). Directly observed treatment of tuberculosis: We can't afford not to try it. *New England Journal of Medicine. 328,* 576–578.

Mundinger, M. (1984, June). Community–based care: Who will be the case managers? *Nursing Outlook 32,* 294–295.

Noble, R.C. (1981). Infectiousness of pulmonary tuberculosis after starting chemotherapy: Review of the available data on an unresolved question. *American Journal of Infection Control, 9,* 6–10.

Poszik, C. J. (1993). Compliance with tuberculosis therapy. *Medical Clinics of North America, 77(6),* 1289–1301.

Reichman, L. B. (1991). The U-shaped curve of concern. *American Review of Respiratory Disease, 144,* 741–742.

Rieder, H. (1993). Case finding. *Lung Biology in Health and Disease, 66,* 167–182.

Sumartojo, E. (1993). When TB treatment fails: A social behavioral account of patient adherence. *American Review of Respiratory Disease, 147,* 1311–1320.

Wolinsky, E. (1993). Statement of the tuberculosis committee of the Infectious Diseases Society of America. *Clinical Infectious Diseases, 16,* 627–628.

PART IV
Special Issues

11

TUBERCULOSIS IN SELECTED POPULATIONS: HIV/AIDS PATIENTS, WOMEN, CHILDREN, AND THE ELDERLY

Felissa L. Cohen, Linda Edwards, Ann E. Kurth, and Elizabeth K. Peabody*

Although tuberculosis (TB) may be acquired by persons at any age, condition, or gender as discussed throughout this book, special aspects deserve consideration. This chapter will consider particular aspects of TB in four groups: persons with human immunodeficiency virus (HIV) infection, women, children, and the elderly.

*Authors are listed alphabetically as equal contributors.

TUBERCULOSIS AND HIV DISEASE

Discussion of TB in relation to HIV-infection and AIDS is integrated in virtually every chapter in this book. Therefore, in order not to be repetitious, only brief information is presented in this chapter. HIV is, at least partly, responsible for the worldwide resurgence of TB and has been called " . . . the most potent risk factor for the development of tuberculosis" (Barnes & Barrows, 1993, p. 400). This association was initially demonstrated by geographic analysis of the overlap of TB and HIV-infection and was confirmed by subsequent prospective studies (Johnson & Chaisson, 1993). In the United States between 1985 and 1990, five states (New York, California, Florida, Texas, and New Jersey) were the top areas for both AIDS cases and increased TB cases. In the United States injecting drug users (IDUs) with HIV-infection are at particular high risk for TB.

   M. tuberculosis infection is endemic in many areas of the world in which HIV-infection is highly prevalent such as sub-Saharan Africa (Horsburgh & Pozniak, 1993). For persons who are infected with *M. tuberculosis* and who also are HIV-infected, the risk for developing tuberculosis is more than 10 times greater than the risk among persons who are HIV-negative and infected with *M. tuberculosis*. In HIV-infected individuals, TB may result from reactivation of previous tuberculous infection (the more common situation) or may be of the primary progressive variety. Outbreaks of TB among HIV-infected persons in group settings have often shown accelerated progression within as few as 3 weeks after exposure (Johnson et al., 1993).

   TB may either precede or follow the diagnosis of HIV-infection and often may be the initial manifestation (Barnes et al., 1993). Extrapulmonary and disseminated TB have long been AIDS-defining condition. Pulmonary TB was added as an AIDS defining disease (coupled with CD4 + counts of < 200 mm^3) in the January 1, 1993, expanded surveillance case definition among adolescents and adults (Centers for Disease Control and Prevention, 1992a). HIV-positive persons should be tested for TB, and persons with TB if appropriate should be tested for HIV (Barnes, Le & Davidson, 1993; Di Ferdinando, Glassroth, Hecht, & Stover, 1993; Pitchenik & Fertel, 1992). Symptoms of TB in a person with HIV-disease is somewhat dependent on immune status and in severe immunosuppression may be atypical. If anergy is present, typical tuberculin testing may not be reactive, and therefore anergy testing should accompany the Mantoux test where appropriate (see Chapter 8). In addition, recommendations for reading the test in those who are HIV-infected are specified (Centers for Disease Control, 1990a; 1991) Symptoms of TB can be similar to some of those found in HIV-disease such as weight loss, cough, anorexia and fever (Johnson et al., 1993; Small & Jacobson, 1994). Extrapulmonary TB is common in those who are HIV-infected and may occur in as many as 70% of the HIV-infected alone or accompany pulmonary TB (Barnes et al., 1993). Chest radiographs may not be typical of TB or may even be normal (Glassroth, 1993). For many reasons, persons who are HIV-infected often acquire multidrug-resistant TB (MDR-TB). The CDC have issued guidelines for the treatment of TB in those who are HIV-infected, and these are discussed in Chapter 5 (Centers for Disease Control and Prevention, 1993a). It has been noted that TB is the only frequent infection in persons with HIV-disease that is transmissible, curable and preventable. These characteristics afford a special opportunity to health-care professionals for action in prevention, education, and treatment.

TUBERCULOSIS IN WOMEN

The image of the pale tuberculosis sufferer was nearly a literary motif of the 19th and early 20th centuries. Charlotte Brönte died of complications from tuberculosis or "consumption", and it was suspected that she may also have been pregnant at the time, though this is speculative (Weiss, 1991). At the turn of the 20th century it was estimated that 1.5% of all pregnant women suffered from clinically symptomatic tuberculosis (Bacon, 1905).

Rates of tuberculosis have increased most dramatically in young adults who are of minority backgrounds and of reproductive-potential ages (Vallejo & Starke, 1992). The return of TB is related to several factors that affect women and children. These include human immunodeficiency virus (HIV) infection; the rise in the number of homeless or unstably housed persons; drug addiction, including crack and cocaine abuse; growing poverty; and a crumbling health infrastructure serving the urban poor (Brudney & Dobkin, 1991).

Poverty and drug addiction are not gender neutral. Women and families comprise an increasing proportion of congregate-living populations, such as in shelters or prisons. The United States has the world's highest known rate of incarceration, with 426 prisoners per 100,000 (Maeur, 1992). Women made up about 3% of the U.S. prison population in 1981; in a little over a decade that proportion has doubled (Harris, 1993, p. 26). One objective of the National Action Plan to Combat MDR-TB (See Appendix 2) is to analyze the incidence and prevalence of tuberculosis in HIV-infected women because little data are now available (Centers for Disease Control, 1992).

Women are among the fastest-growing group of persons with HIV disease. Nurses and other health care professionals must be alert to the possibility of TB cases in vulnerable populations, including women and children (Kurth, 1993). This section will describe issues regarding screening, prophylaxis, HIV disease, and treatment concerns for women.

Epidemiology

The number of cases of TB occurring in U.S. women in 1992 was 9,238 or nearly 40% of all reported cases (Centers for Disease Control and Prevention, 1993c). In U.S. women of childbearing age, the reported number of TB cases increased about 41% between 1985 and 1992 (Cantwell, et al., 1994). It was estimated that in 1992 nearly half of all new HIV infections around the world occurred in women (Merson, 1992). In the United States, the majority of women with HIV infection are nonwhite and in the reproductive-potential years, paralleling the peak years for tuberculosis cases in the nonwhite group. It is important to point out that up to one-third of all TB cases are identified among those not in lower socioeconomic groups, and practitioners should be careful not to make assumptions about a given patient's HIV or TB risks. Studies conducted among women in Zaire and Rwanda showed that the annual TB risk for HIV-positive women was 28 to 31 times higher than for HIV-negative women (Narain, Raviglione, & Kochi, 1992).

Pregnancy and Tuberculosis

Although more rarely encountered in developed countries, primary infection or reactivation of TB during parturition can occur. However, TB is increasing in pregnant women in the United States, particularly in areas where TB is epidemic. In one New York City hospital, the case rate was 12.4 per 100,000 deliveries from 1985-1992. From 1991-1992, the case rate was 94.8 per 100,000 deliveries (Margono, Mroueh, Garely et al., 1994). Many experts feel that the rate of TB activation in women who are tuberculin test reactors is not changed by pregnancy itself (Witter, 1988). Others, however, point out that pregnancy suppresses cell-mediated immunity, which may predispose a woman to reactivation of previous tuberculous infection, or possibly to new exogenous tuberculous infection (Warner, Khoo, & Wilkins, 1992).

Historical opinion on the effect of pregnancy on tuberculosis outcome has varied. As late as 1835, some physicians felt that pregnancy had a beneficial effect; however, by the mid-19th century pregnancy was felt to be so adverse to the prognosis for women with tuberculosis that abortions were routinely recommended. Today, the prevailing feeling is that, given adequate treatment for active tuberculosis, pregnant women should have prognoses that are equivalent to their nonpregnant counterparts (Burrow & Ferris, 1988; Snider, 1984). In summary, no conclusive evidence exists that pregnancy itself has an adverse effect on the course of adequately treated tuberculosis (Burrow & Ferris, 1988; Snider, 1984).

Any woman who receives prenatal care should be screened for tuberculous infection and disease and effective treatment instituted if necessary. Studies have shown that many pregnant women (19–60%) with active TB may present asymptomatically or with symptoms that mimic normal physiologic changes of pregnancy (Hamadeh, & Glassroth, 1992; Witter, 1988). Thus, Mantoux testing (as described in Chapter 8) is a standard part of antepartal care. Case-controlled studies have shown that pregnancy does not affect delayed-type hypersensitivity reactions; thus tuberculin testing should be valid throughout pregnancy (Snider, 1984). Approximately 1 to 2 percent of pregnant women in urban indigent areas and up to 15 to 25 percent of women from Southeast Asia will show reactivity on the tuberculin skin test (Bowes, 1987).

Chest radiography with abdominal shielding is indicated in those reactors who have recently converted or in whom the date of conversion is unknown, and in those women with a suggestive history, symptoms, or physical findings (Burrows et al., 1988). If possible, the chest radiograph should be done after the first trimester, particularly if no symptoms are present (Centers for Disease Control and Prevention, 1993b; Mays, 1993). Sputum samples for both smear and culture (including drug sensitivity testing) should be obtained immediately in those who are reactive on skin testing or have other positive findings (see Chapters 4 & 8) (Witter, 1988). The diaphragmatic compression of the lungs seen as pregnancy advances can mask actual pulmonary cavitation. For this reason, initiation of treatment in a pregnant woman may need to be undertaken with less evidence than in a nonpregnant woman (Pritchard, MacDonald, and Gant, 1985).

Some women receive no prenatal care at all for various reasons that can include impaired access, immigration status, addiction, and fear of medical services. Beyond the obvious risks of untreated tuberculosis to the woman herself and to the fetus due to compromised oxygenation, other obstetrical complications can arise. For example, a persistent, vigorous cough may lead to abortion, premature labor, or premature separation of the placenta in the third stage of labor, resulting in hemorrhage (Ajayi, 1980).

Intrapartal analgesia and anesthesia methods used during normal pregnancies can be used for the women with tuberculosis as long as pulmonary function is not seriously impaired and delivery by standard methods is usual (Hamadeh, & Glassroth, 1992; Pritchard et al., 1985).

If the antepartal tuberculin test is negative, assuming the woman has no evidence of cutaneous anergy, no further evaluation is needed. In the case of a reactive tuberculin test when the physical examination and chest radiographs are negative, and active TB is not present, chemoprophylaxis is not usually started until after delivery. However, as stated earlier, in certain populations such as women with HIV-disease, the risk of TB progression is such that prophylaxis may be started immediately. Preventive therapy should be evaluated on a case-to-case basis (Centers for Disease Control and Prevention, 1994b).

When treatment is required during pregnancy, several considerations apply. Despite the usual concerns about administering drugs during pregnancy, the risk of untreated active TB is such that treatment is warranted and the recommended initial regimen is isoniazid (INH), rifampin and ethambutol for 9 months (Centers for Disease Control and Prevention, 1993a). One extensive review of the literature (Snider, Layde, Johnson, & Lyle, 1980) found that only 2.89% of fetuses exposed to INH, rifampin, ethambutol, or para-aminosalicylic acid were classified as having birth defects, a rate that does not differ appreciably from that for all births. Pyridoxine 50 mg (B_6) should be given to the woman taking INH because, in addition to other reasons, B_6 can minimize the potential for neurotoxicities in the fetus as well as satisfy the increased need during pregnancy (Atkins, 1982; Burrow et al., 1988). Because of their teratogenicity or limited safety data, streptomycin, pyrazinamide, the aminoglycosides, capreomycin, ciprofloxacin, ofloxacin, ethionamide, cycloserine, and clofazimine should all be avoided during pregnancy (Frieden & Fujiwara, 1992). General treatment regimens and drugs are discussed in Chapter 5.

Congenital and Neonatal Tuberculosis

Congenital tuberculous infection is uncommon. Transmission can occur through aspiration or ingestion of infected amniotic fluid or through hematogenous spread (Burrow et al., 1988; Cantwell et al., 1994; Mudido & Speck, 1994: Rosenfeld, Hageman & Yogev, 1993). Perinatal TB may also be acquired during the birth process from aspiration or ingestion if the mother has endocervical TB (Mudido & Speck, 1994; Rosenfeld, Hageman & Yogev, 1993). Symptoms are usually nonspecific but may be seen in the first month of life. The most commonly seen manifestations of congenital TB are fever, respiratory distress, hepatomegaly, splenomegaly, poor feeding, poor weight gain, lethargy, and irritability (Mudido & Speck, 1994).

Recently, revised criteria for distinguishing between congenital and postnatally acquired TB have been proposed (Cantwell, et al., 1994). The 25 to 35% of children born to HIV-positive mothers who are themselves truly HIV-infected may also be at risk for TB because of immunosuppression (De Cock, Soro, Coulibaly, & Lucas 1992). In developing countries, the World Health Organization (WHO) recommends that newborns of known or suspected HIV-positive mothers should be given the Bacille Calmette-Guérin (BCG) vaccination (Narain et al., 1992). The WHO recommends though that the BCG should be withheld from persons with symptomatic HIV- disease or those living in countries where the risk of TB is low (De Cock, et al., 1992). The use of BCG for tuberculosis prevention has long been controversial in general, and the safety and efficacy of BCG in HIV-infected persons is not established at this time (Weltman & Rose, 1993).

If a woman is identified with active TB only after delivery, some believe that the infant should be isolated until the mother is not infectious. However, bonding may be affected. Some have pointed out that even with AFB-negative sputum smears, there may still be a risk of maternal transmission (Sweet & Brown, 1991). Several options for medical regimens are available, depending on the context and probability of treatment adherence. One is to prophylactically treat the infant from birth with INH at 10 to 20 mg/kg/day for 9 months, or until the mother and other household contacts are documented to be noninfective (Bowes, 1987). Another is to vaccinate the infant with BCG if the infant is not actively infected (Burrow et al., 1988).

Tuberculosis and Breast-feeding

Breast milk of mothers with pulmonary tuberculosis has been found to contain some TB bacilli, though it is not seen as a transmission source (Chebotareva, 1990). However, lactating mothers with active tuberculosis should be receiving chemotherapy to prevent respiratory spread to the infant. INH can be excreted in breast milk and thus poses some risk of hepatotoxicity in the infant, leading some to recommend that breast-feeding is contraindicated in women receiving anti-TB therapies (Berkowitz, et al., 1986). However, other experts have estimated that no more than 20% of the usual therapeutic dose for infants is actually excreted in breast milk, thus leading to the conclusion that the risk of drug toxicity to nursing infants is quite low (Snider, 1984). Breast-feeding during tuberculosis treatment should, therefore, not be discouraged (Hamadeh et al., 1992), with the understanding that drug levels in the breast milk are not sufficient to prevent or treat TB in the newborn (Frieden et al., 1992) and that the infant may need supplemental pyridoxine (Witter, 1988). If the infant is already receiving anti-TB treatment, the infant should be observed for toxicity, or the discontinuance of breast-feeding should be considered. Partial bottle feeding may be a solution (Hamadeh et al., 1992).

Special Treatment Considerations in Women

Tuberculosis treatment of women is not different from that of men unless the woman is pregnant. Whether a patient adheres to a treatment regimen or not can be influenced by a number of factors, which may in some cases be influenced by gender. Generally, patient characteristics such as gender have not consistently been shown to affect adherence; however it has been pointed out that access to health services does. Workers in lower paying jobs (e.g., waitressing) often don't have sick leave. This means that coming to TB clinics costs both time and money (Snider & Hutton, 1989). Women who are unemployed may not have the means for transportation and thus may be more focused on higher priority survival issues such as food and housing. Finally, those women who are active drug users often have little incentive to access the health care system. For those women, who are often the sole caretakers and who may be sick, adhering to appointment schedules for either herself or her children can be very difficult. Creative solutions on the part of the health care provider may require finding transportation and/or childcare in these situations (see Chapter 8).

Tuberculosis and Gynecological Considerations

Tuberculous salpingitis accounts for a small percentage of all pelvic inflammatory disease (PID) and its sequelae in the United States (Wynn, 1988). Although relatively rare in the United States, it is frequent in other parts of the world, and should be considered as a cause of PID in women who have recently immigrated from Asia, the Middle East, or Latin America (Herbst, Mishell, Stenchever, & Droegemueller, 1992). Tuberculous PID results from disseminated spread of tuberculosis to the ovary, Fallopian tubes, and the endometrium. The Fallopian tube is often the primary site of infection, destroying the fimbria and eliminating peristalsis. Symptoms are often nonspecific, including malaise, low-grade fever, and persistent abdominal pain; menstrual disorders and infertility often ensue. Tuberculosis should be ruled out in any case of salpingitis that does not respond to standard treatment or in the case of PID in women with no history of sexual intercourse.

The majority of women with tuberculous salpingitis also have tuberculous endometritis, and some may have urinary tract TB. Diagnosis is confirmed by testing of endometrial biopsy specimens and a work-up for urinary tract TB should also be done. Early, aggressive chemotherapy may be warranted to salvage fertility in at least some patients (Durukan, Urman, Yarali, Arikan, & Beykal, 1990; Herbst et al., 1992). Administration of anti-tuberculous drugs for 9 to 24 months is the treatment of choice. Surgical treatment is generally used only for those with persistent pelvic masses and for those whose endometrial cultures remain positive (Herbst et al., 1992; Wynn, 1988).

TUBERCULOSIS AND CHILDREN

The rates of childhood TB in the United States declined between 1962 and 1987 but began to increase in 1988. Of the reported cases in 1988, those under 5 years of age accounted for approximately 60%. Seven states (California, Florida, Georgia, Illinois, New York, South Carolina, and Texas) accounted for more than 60% of the reported cases, and metropolitan areas of 250,000 or more reported the highest pediatric TB rates (Jacobs & Starke, 1993). Other age-related epidemiology is discussed in Chapter 3.

When TB occurs in children, it is significant because infection in children represents recent transmission and thus is a "marker" for transmission in other age groups and a reservoir for future cases (Agrons, Markowitz & Kramer, 1993; Starke, 1993). Nearly all infection in children occurs through contact with active disease among household members; in fact, "each case of tuberculosis in young children represents failure of identification of contacts and preventive measures" (Nemir & Krasinski, 1988, p. 377). TB has been called a family disease because TB-infected children commonly have a TB-infected parent(s) (Bakshi, et al., 1993). It is equally important to keep in mind that children are the reservoirs from which future cases will be transmitted (Starke, 1988; Starke & Kym, 1989). Infants and children are at high risk of TB infection when

1. a family member is infected with HIV;
2. a family member is infected with TB;
3. the family has recently immigrated from a country with high tuberculosis rates;

4. they are numbered among the homeless and/or migrant populations (Bakshi, et al., 1993; Engel, 1989; Feigin & Cherry, 1992; Lanphear & Snider, 1991).
5. they have another condition that puts them at risk such as HIV infection, immunosuppressive conditions, chronic renal failure, malnutrition, diabetes mellitus, Hodgkin's disease or lymphoma; and
6. they are frequently exposed to adults who inject drugs, have infectious TB, are poor city dwellers, are migrant farm workers, or are residents of institutions such as nursing homes (Bakski, et al., 1993; Committee on Infectious Diseases, 1994; Engel, 1989; Feigin & Cherry, 1992; Lanphear & Snider, 1991).

It is particularly alarming, then, to note that families with children are the fastest growing segment of homeless persons (Oberg, 1991). In addition to homelessness, children in urban settings may be living in crowded, unhealthy conditions that also can predispose to TB (Drucker, Alcabes, Bosworth & Sckell 1994).

Age also is significantly related to the development of active disease. Infants are susceptible to *Mycobacterium tuberculosis* because of decreased overall resistance and a lack of ability to localize infection (Richardson, Zickler & Wheat, 1991). Risk of infection and subsequent active disease is greatest among children under 2 years of age because of underdeveloped immune systems. Children younger than 5 years of age have twice the risk of developing active disease as those who are older than 5 years (American Thoracic Society, 1990; Dowling, 1991). One study of children who were tuberculin reactors found that 83 percent of those under 3 years of age had active tuberculosis (Nemir et al., 1988).

Children from 5 to 14 years are generally viewed as at lower risk than either older or younger children. Nevertheless, when infected with TB, children in this age group bear an undue burden of disease; because of the asymptomatic nature of tuberculosis in children from 5 through 14, cases are likely to be severe and often have progressed to pulmonary cavitations by the time they are found at adolescence (Nemir et al., 1988).

As children mature to puberty, their risk of infection is again increased. The mechanism of this phenomenon, whether due to increased contact opportunities because of the adolescent's expanding world, or to hormonal changes, dietary fads, or a combination of these is unclear (Richardson et al., 1991). Even previously treated, well-supervised, adherent children may have reactivation of disease at adolescence (Nemir, 1986). Incarcerated adolescents or those who inject drugs are at particularly high risk for TB infection (Committee on Infectious Diseases, 1994).

Another dimension of childhood tuberculosis is the increase in numbers of childless couples who are adopting foreign-born children. Many of these children may have suffered prolonged periods of deprivation. Often little is known about their preadoption medical history. A recent study of 293 foreign born-children arriving in the United States for adoption revealed that 3% had reactive tuberculin tests with induration of 10 mm or larger. Only 1 out of 10 had a history of receiving BCG vaccine (or a recognizable scar). Four children had active tuberculosis (Hostetter et al., 1991).

In elementary and high school grades, girls have a much higher incidence of tuberculosis than boys (Feigin et al., 1992). Known factors that increase risk of infection include other chronic illnesses, undernutrition, emotional stress, and chronic fatigue (Richardson et al., 1991). These factors are often more prevalent in those who are socioeconomically disadvantaged.

Characteristics of Tuberculosis in Children

One of the major difficulties in detecting TB in children is that nearly half of infants and as many as 90 to 95% of older children with active disease have no specific symptoms (Richardson et al., 1991) or may be asymptomatic (Jacobs & Eisenach Jacobs et al., 1993). As a result, at-risk children with vague health complaints should be assessed for tuberculosis, especially when there is chronic cough, wheezing, perihilar adenopathy and/or obstructive airway (Oberg, 1991; Richardson et al., 1991). Chest radiography may also be important in the diagnosis of TB in children (Agrons, Markowitz & Kramer, 1993).

The vast majority of children with tuberculosis (92%) have lung or lymph node involvement; however, the adenitis found with tuberculosis may mimic other diseases, particularly those with nontubercular mycobacteria (Snider et al., 1988). Although the primary lesion may be similar to that in adults, children are more likely than adults to develop extrapulmonary disease, which is seen in approximately 25% of children under the age of 4 years (Jacobs et al., 1993). Cervical lymphadenitis is one of the most common forms of extrapulmonary TB in children. Other common sites seen in childhood are bone, joint, central nervous system (usually meningeal), and the abdomen. Genitourinary disease is seen in adolescents (Jacobs et al., 1993; McIntosh et al., 1993). Miliary (disseminated) TB is a relatively common complication in young children and occurs significantly more frequently than among adults. The miliary form of tuberculosis in children has a very high mortality rate. An early complication of miliary disease found in infants and young children is tuberculous meningitis. This may have vague symptoms at first, such as personality changes, listlessness and anorexia, followed by headache, vomiting, and a rigid neck (Feigen et al., 1992; Jacobs & Starke, 1993) In some cases, this complication appears to be precipitated by a viral infection, a fall, or a blow to the head (Feigin et al., 1992).

HIV-Infection and Tuberculosis in Children

HIV infection impacts on TB in children in a variety of ways. Children who are HIV-infected, like adults, are at higher risk of developing TB than are their non-HIV-infected counterparts (Bakshi et al., 1993). In New York City, children with symptomatic HIV-disease were reported to have a rate of TB that was 10 times higher than that of all children in New York City (Lyon, Thomas, Caldwell, & Admassur, 1992). In addition, HIV-infected children are more likely to develop symptomatic TB than are non-HIV-infected children, even within the same family. They are more likely to have progressive primary disease than are adults. If an adult in a family with an HIV-infected child develops TB, then isoniazid prophylaxis, given to the child for a period of 6 to 12 months (and with the addition of rifampin if the strain is resistant to isoniazid), may be useful in prevention (See Chapter 5). Children living with HIV-infected adults should be screened frequently (every 6 to 12 months) by use of the Mantoux tuberculin test (Bakshi et al., 1993). A further consideration is that TB is one of the few infections acquired by children with HIV-disease that can put others (such as health care workers and teachers) at risk of acquisition of TB. Nurses working in settings where HIV-infected children are present should be aware of subtle changes that could indicate TB infection.

Impact of Aggregate Settings

Because of the close contact and proximity of children and adults in schools, day care centers, and other aggregate settings, nurses working in these locations need to give special considerations to factors implicit in the natural history of TB. Outbreaks have been known to occur in these settings, usually resulting to exposure to adults who are infected with TB. Children who are in active stages of disease are less likely to be infectious to others than are adults because they lack tussive force to their cough, are more likely to have a nonproductive cough, and have fewer active organisms in endobronchial secretions; however transmission from children can occur, and infectiousness should be evaluated in the same way as in adults, particularly for isolation precautions (Centers for Disease Control and Prevention, 1994b; Feigin & Cherry, 1992; Smith, 1989; Starke, 1988). Although the need for isolation is rare, families may feel stigmatized and socially isolated if one of the children or other members has active TB. The nurse can help the individual family and provide educational assistance through the schools. Although children with active disease rarely infect other children, the lack of clearly defined symptomatology, particularly in early stages, may result in children with TB going undetected and untreated, thus progressing to later disease stages before diagnosis (Smith, 1989). Consequently, schools and other aggregate settings deserve special attention.

The earlier declines in incidence among children have given communities a false sense of security; many areas in the United States subsequently have elected to discontinue school requirements for tuberculin testing (Starke, 1988). Other countries have not followed this example and continue to require screening tests prior to school entrance. England, for instance, has mandated tuberculin testing as part of the required school medical examination since 1955 (Miller & Thompson, 1992).

Current recommendations for screening among children include tuberculin testing of selected high-risk populations, rather than routine screening of all children (Committee on Infectious Diseases, 1994; Snider et al, 1988). Screening of school children from high-risk populations is viewed as a most successful method of determining those who are infected and in need of treatment and/or prophylaxis (Schutze, Rice, & Starke, 1993). This screening (with the Mantoux test) can be done when the child enters elementary school and upon entry to high school (Feigin et al., 1992; Nemir & O'Hare, 1991). The American Academy of Pediatrics has recommended that children at high risk for TB should be skin tested annually. Those children with no risk factors or incomplete or unreliable histories, and those who reside in high TB prevalence areas may be tested periodically at such ages as 1 year, between 4 and 6 years, and between 11 and 16 years of age. This testing (using the Mantoux test) should be based on the local epidemiology of TB (Committee on Infectious Diseases, 1994). TB in adolescents can result easily in cavitation and positive sputum, making them infectious to others. Detecting conversions by means of the Mantoux test can allow early therapy and contact tracing (see Chapters 8 and 10) (Nemir & O'Hare, 1991).

Nursing Implications

School nurses, including community health nurses who serve children in any aggregate setting, are an important part of the network of services needed to prevent, identify, and treat tuberculosis among children. These nurses are critical in implementing control efforts at all levels of prevention, including health promotion.

Health Promotion. Efforts in schools to develop healthier lifestyles among children and adolescents impact on students' abilities to withstand the disease process and minimize exposure. Children who are taught good nutrition, stress management, proper rest and fitness measures, and good hygiene and health consumer skills are more likely to reduce their risk of contracting disease and/or resist active infection (Richardson et al., 1991).

Primary Prevention. Specific protective measures that school nurses can institute include appropriate screening of school personnel who come in close contact with children for TB and health education. As with school requirements for children, requirements for screening school personnel also decreased when this country became more complacent about tuberculosis. Education pertinent to TB should be incorporated into health education classes (Nemir, 1986). Also, because children are often the only entrée to some families, informational materials specific to tuberculosis can be sent to homes and frequently will impact on family members and friends.

Policy makers may consider other specific protective measures and seek clarification about BCG vaccine as a preventive strategy for children. School nurses and community health nurses can have input into decisions affecting use of the vaccine. Studies of BCG administered to children have demonstrated protection ranging from 17 to 90% (Snider et al., 1988). Because the protective power is so variable, the vaccine is not seen as a reliable method of preventing tuberculosis in the United States (Nemir et al., 1988). In spite of this variability in shielding against infection, there is evidence that demonstrates protection for children against the more severe complications of tuberculosis, namely, tuberculous meningitis and miliary tuberculosis (Hussey, Chisholm, & Kebel, 1991; Snider, et al., 1988). At this time, BCG is only recommended as an alternative when children who are not infected are at unavoidable risk of exposure (Dowling, 1991). It should not be given to children who are immunocompromised ("Use of BCG", 1988). BCG is further discussed in Chapter 5.

Secondary Prevention. The school nurse's role in secondary prevention is instrumental and many faceted. Reviews of health history information gathered during physical examinations, special education evaluations, and individual contacts with students and parents provide information for identifying children at risk and in early stages of disease. The nurse can utilize health histories to identify parents and grandparents from any of the high-risk groups (Feigin et al., 1992).

Among the potential reservoirs of infection at home are household members who are HIV-infected. (Khouri, Mastrucci, Hutto, Mitchell, & Scott, 1992). In addition, children who are infected with both HIV and tuberculosis often do not evidence a positive tuberculin test because of anergy (see Chapter 8) (Khouri et al., 1992). Since progression of tuberculosis may be atypical in children who are immunosuppressed because of HIV-infection, cancer, or chronic illness, nurses in child care and educational facilities must be alert to relatively unnoticeable changes in health status. These immunosuppressed children, if infected with *M. tuberculosis*, are more likely to develop miliary tuberculosis (DeHaan & Benson, 1992). Another group targeted for special concern are pregnant adolescents who have tuberculous infection or TB (Nemir, 1986).

Children who are tuberculin tested by health care providers often fail to return for reading of the test results. In most cases, reliance is placed upon the parent or guardian to check the child's arm, make an accurate assessment, and report the results to the health provider. School nurses can play a valuable role in assessing the results of testing and providing a confident report to the primary provider. When screening is conducted at school, responsibility is placed on the nurse for following through on evaluation of the test results. False negatives may occur with several diseases of childhood, including measles, mumps, and chicken pox, as well as with live virus vaccines (Dowling, 1991).

The school nurse also can assist in improving adherence with treatment routines, whether for prophylaxis or for active disease. Although newer and shorter regimens are being instituted, adherence remains an issue (Abernathy, Jacobs, & Stead, 1991; Engel, 1989; Starke et al., 1989). The nurse can assist children on medication with adherence by involving families in the treatment plan and by working with them to set mutual goals and convenient follow-up schedules (Richardson et al., 1991). In some instances, the school nurse can be utilized for "directly observed therapy" (DOT) confirmation (Engel, 1989). DOT is discussed in Chapters 7 and 10.

Occasionally, school nurses may be requested to assist in collecting specimens for diagnostic or evaluative tests. Accurate information on effective procedures for use with children will assist in timely collections (American Thoracic Society, 1990).

During early months of treatment, the nurse can assist children to safeguard health by avoiding overfatigue, competitive sports, excessive study, sunburn, and stressful situations. Following this initial period, children with active tuberculosis need not have activity limitations while in school unless pulmonary symptoms (e.g., shortness of breath) preclude strenuous activity (Feigin et al., 1992).

Tertiary Prevention. Long-term sequellae from successfully treated tuberculosis are rare, unless complicated by damage to the central nervous system, such as occurs with tuberculous meningitis. Often, though, the nurse needs to be aware of potential complications and/or side effects resulting from the medications used in treatment. In addition, the presence of unrelieved and unaddressed side effects may contribute to nonadherence and noncompletion of the proper therapy. The drug therapy for TB for both adults and children is discussed in detail in Chapter 5, and adherence is discussed in Chapter 7. Isoniazid and rifampin can interact with Dilantin (Dowling, 1991), which is relevant because many children of school age use Dilantin for seizure control. School children with asthma who are medicated with theophylline and isoniazid and/or rifampin may need their dosage of theophylline adjusted because of interactions (Richardson et al, 1991). The school nurse is a key person in identifying these instances, because physicians treating the TB may not be aware of other chronic illnesses.

Since ethambutol can cause toxicity to the optic nerve, it is rarely used with children; however, as bacterial strains that are resistant to preferred drugs become more frequent, there may be children receiving ethambutol who need vision monitoring for acuity and color vision to detect early optic damage (Feigin et al., 1992; Richardson et al., 1991; Snider, et al., 1988). In one Texas study (Starke et al., 1989), these tests were performed monthly. If the child is receiving streptomycin as treatment, then hearing should be monitored regularly because hearing loss can be a side effect (Starke, 1988). Taking rifampin may be particularly difficult (it may scare or embarrass them) for children or adolescents because of its property of turning body fluids reddish orange. Rifampin interacts with many medications (See Chapter 5). Sexually active adolescent girls need to use birth control other than oral contraceptives if taking rifampin.

A key aspect of the school and community health nurses' role in pediatric tuberculosis is the ongoing coordination of multiple facets of care in group settings, based on expert knowledge and practice. It is important that health professionals communicate with each other regarding families affected by tuberculosis.

THE ELDERLY AND TUBERCULOSIS

When all U.S. TB cases are considered without regard to race, the 65 years and older group is highest in case numbers, percent distribution, and TB case rates per 100,000 population. When race is examined with age, TB cases in the United States have the greatest *raw number* and *percent distribution* in the 65 year and older group in the white population. In the nonwhite population, the raw number and percent distribution is highest for the 35-to-44-year-old and 25-to-34-year-old groups. However, the TB case *rate* per 100,000 population for persons 65 years and older is higher than for any other age grouping for both whites and non-whites (Centers for Disease Control and Prevention, 1994a). These distributions are shown in Figures 11.1 and 11.2. In the 65 years of age and older group, males are affected more than females in both the raw number of cases and the case rate, but not in the percent distribution of cases within each gender group. In the percent distribution of cases within each gender, a higher percentage of cases occurs for females of all races in the 65 years and older group. Among the elderly, TB case rates per 100,000 are highest in nonwhite males (111.2) followed by nonwhite females (44.2), white males (18.9) and white females (8.8) (Centers for Disease Control and Prevention, 1994). In all of these statistics, those with HIV-disease are included in the data.

When race is not considered, the incidence of TB in persons over 65 years of age is thus higher than any other population group, except those who are HIV-infected, and TB case rates are higher in those over 65 years of age than any other age group (Dutt & Stead, 1993; McDonald, 1993). Although the elderly account for about 26% of the total U.S.-reported TB cases, this age group represents only 12.5% of the U. S. population (Centers for Disease Control, 1990b; 1994a).

The predominant cause of TB in the elderly is reactivation of an old latent infection acquired many years earlier. As discussed in Chapter 3, 50 to 70 years ago the majority of elderly Americans had been infected with *Mycobacterium tuberculosis* by the age of 30 years. The persistence of that infection is said to account for 90% of the TB cases that occur in elderly persons (Dutt & Stead, 1992; Stead & Dutt, 1991). Factors that increase the risk for endogenous reactivation of a previous TB infection and that may be seen in the elderly include emotional stress, alcoholism, malnutrition, gastrectomy, poorly controlled diabetes mellitus, chronic renal failure, prolonged corticosteroid therapy, immunosuppressive therapy, and malignancies (American Thoracic Society, 1994; Wolinsky, 1992; Yoshikawa, 1992). Further, old age in and of itself may result in a diminished cell-mediated immune response, allowing both endogenous reactivation and exogenous acquisition to occur. Aging T-lymphocytes may have decreased the ability to produce interleukin-2 among other defects (McDonald, 1993; Yoshikawa, 1992). Elderly persons often lose their ability to respond immunologically to the standard tuberculin skin test as discussed in Chapter 8. The findings of Dorken,

216   Special Issues

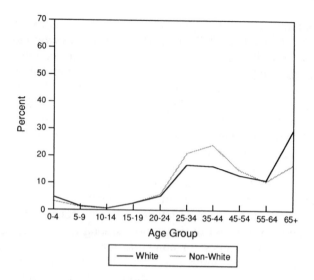

FIGURE 11.1 Percent distribution of tuberculosis cases by age and race, 1992.

Source: Centers for Disease Control. (1994a). *1992 tuberculosis statistics in the United States*. Atlanta, GA: U.S. Department of Health and Human Services.

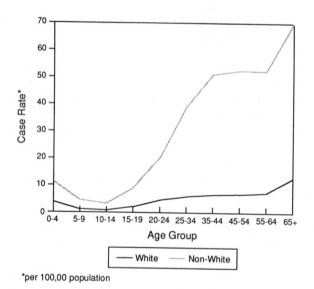

*per 100,00 population

FIGURE 11.2 Tuberculosis cases rates by age and race, 1992.

Source:; Centers for Disease Control. (1994a). *1992 tuberculosis statistics in the United States*. Atlanta, GA: U.S. Department of Health and Human Services.

Grzybowski and Allen (1987) showed that the prevalence of tuberculin skin test reactivity was higher in men than in women in each age group. The reactivity also fell appreciably in both sexes as age increased. In men aged 65 to 74 years, reactivity was 50%, declining to 10.5% in men over 95 years. In women aged 65 to 74 years, reactivity was 36.5%, declining to 8.2% in women over 95 years.

Tuberculosis has low infectivity among casual contacts. Its infectivity is higher among long-term household contacts and in those sharing closed environments such as nursing homes or shelters for the homeless. Stead (1981) described an epidemic of tuberculosis in a nursing home in which one 72-year-old resident with active tuberculosis infected 49 residents. Eight residents developed progressive primary tuberculosis with one subsequent death. The epidemic was finally stopped by treating all tuberculin skin test converters with isoniazid.

In one comparison of annual incidence rates of TB among the elderly, it was found that the rate was 39.2 per 100,000 population for those in nursing homes as compared with 21.5 per 100,000 population for those living in the community (Centers for Disease Control, 1990). In Arkansas, in 1985, it was reported that the TB case rate was 17 per 100,000 in the general population; 60 per 100,000 in those over age 65 years living at home, and 234 per 100,000 in those over age 65 years living in a nursing home (Dutt et al., 1993). Thus, it is important that tuberculin testing be done on entry to the nursing home or long-term care facility, with follow-up of reactors to be rule out active TB (Dutt et al., 1992). Failure to identify TB cases in nursing homes can result in the spread of infection to other residents, volunteers, and staff.

Guidelines and Recommendations for Long-Term Care Facilities

The CDC have made recommendations for surveillance, containment, assessment, education, and control for TB for use by long-term care facilities and nursing homes (Centers for Disease Control, 1990). The major recommendations are shown in Table 11.1. Staff employed in nursing homes and facilities should be tuberculin skin tested on employment with the two-step method (Dutt et al., 1993). In this method, a second Mantoux test is done within 1 to 2 weeks of a negative initial test to increase the detection of true positive responses because of the booster effect (see Chapter 8 and following section) (Yoshikawa, 1992). Preventive therapy should be considered for those who are reactors as discussed in the guidelines in Chapter 5. Staff members have less of a risk of tuberculin skin test conversion than the residents in a nursing home or long term care facility because the time they spend in the facility is less than that spent by the residents (Dutt et al., 1993).

TABLE 11.1 Major Recommendations For The Prevention and Control of Tuberculosis in Facilities Providing Long-Term Care to the Elderly

Surveillance — identifying and reporting all TB cases in the facility with appropriate institution of therapy.
- Tuberculin skin testing by the Mantoux method using 5 units of PPD should be administered to:
  all new residents on admission
  new employees at the time of employment
  volunteers with resident contact of 10 or more hours per week
- The two-step method should be used for residents and employees and results should be documented in medical records or personnel files.
- All persons with a tuberculin skin test reaction of 10 mm or more should receive a chest radiograph to identify current or past tuberculosis, and further testing or treatment as needed.
- Repeat tuberculin testing should be done for negative employees, residents or volunteers depending on the risk of tuberculous infection in the particular facility, and should be provided after a suspected exposure to a case of active TB.
- Each skin test converter (defined as an increase of 10 or more mm for a person 35 years of age or younger or an increase of 15 or more mm for a person 35 years of age or older) should have a chest radiograph. Further management and testing depends on the results. If it is negative, they should receive preventive treatment.
- Staff members considered to have infectious TB should be relieved of work responsibilities until diagnosis is excluded or until they become noninfectious.
- Suspected or confirmed TB should be appropriately recorded in the records and the local or state health department should be notified in accordance with the laws or regulations of that state.
- Staff members and residents with tuberculous infection or tuberculosis should be assessed for HIV infection with appropriate counseling and testing.
Containment — ensures that transmission of TB is promptly stopped.
- Persons with suspected or confirmed tuberculosis can remain in their usual environment, provided 1) chemotherapy is promptly instituted at the time the diagnosis is suspected or confirmed, 2) recent and current contacts are evaluated and placed on appropriate therapy, and 3) new contacts can be prevented for a 1- to 2-week period. If these conditions can be met, the person with suspected or confirmed tuberculosis should be placed under appropriate isolation precautions to prevent the spread of the infections.
- Treatment recommendations of the American Thoracic Society/Centers for Disease Control should be followed in treating and managing persons with confirmed or suspected tuberculosis
- "Close contacts," defined as persons who sleep, live, work, or who are otherwise in close contact with an infectious person through a common ventilation system for a prolonged time are at risk of acquiring TB infection. These persons may include other residents, staff, and visitors. When a person with confirmed tuberculosis appears to be infectious, contacts who were previously tuberculin-negative should be retested. If the case occurs in a known tuberculin converter, the source case should be identified.

Table 11.1, continued

- General guidelines for conducting a contact investigation in a nursing home or other facility are given in the appendix to the report.
- Preventive therapy guidelines are summarized in the report but have recently been updated and current information should be sought (Centers for Disease Control and Prevention, 1993a).

Assessment — monitoring and evaluating the surveillance and containment activities.

- A careful record keeping system is essential for tracking and assessing the status of persons with TB in facilities that provide long-term care for elderly persons. The document specifies data that should be kept and reviewed with the health department staff.

Education — refers to providing information and imparting skills to patients, visitors, and employees so that they understand and cooperate with surveillance, containment, and assessment activities.

Role of the Health Department

- State and local health departments should assist in developing and updating policies, procedures, and record systems for TB control in facilities that provide residential care for elderly persons.
- They should provide access to expert TB medical consultation and assistance in investigations of contacts and management of outbreaks in the facility.
- They should maintain a TB registry.
- The health department should train facility staff to administer, read, and record tuberculin skin tests, identify signs and symptoms of TB, initiate and observe therapy, monitor for side effects, collect diagnostic specimens, and maintain record systems.

Source: Centers for Disease Control (1990). Prevention and control of tuberculosis in facilities providing long-term care to the elderly. Recommendations of the Advisory Committee for Elimination of Tuberculosis. *Morbidity and Mortality Weekly Report, 39(RR-10),* 7–13.

Clinical Manifestations and Assessment In The Elderly

Tuberculosis may involve any organ system, but the lung is the usual site of the primary lesion and the principal organ involved in the elderly as in all age groups (Wolinsky, 1992). Pulmonary TB in younger populations may present with the symptoms of a productive cough and/or non-specific symptoms such as fever, anorexia, weight loss, night sweats or chills, weakness and malaise (Schluger & Rom, 1994; Wolinsky, 1988). Sometimes there are no specific symptoms. In the elderly, often the symptoms presented can be explained by a variety of other medical problems commonly encountered, or symptoms may be absent or atypical. Misdiagnosis is particularly frequent when TB complicates lung cancer or chronic obstructive pulmonary disease in an elderly person (Couser & Glassroth, 1993; McDonald, 1993). Chest radiographic features that are typical of TB may be different in the elderly. The picture can include diffuse miliary infiltrates or fibronodular infiltrates in the upper lung zones or the superior segment of the lower lobes. Sometimes TB is misdiagnosed as pneumonia. In cases where the person is recently infected with TB that has progressed to active disease and is thus primary, the radiographic abnormalities may be seen in the middle and lower lung zones. New primary TB in the elderly may be manifested as pleural effusion and mistaken for congestive heart failure (Dutt et al., 1992; McDonald, 1993; Moulding, 1994).

Extrapulmonary TB occurs in the elderly as well as younger age groups. The most frequent sites seen are miliary TB (disseminated widely), renal, pericardium, vertebra, or meninges. In meningeal TB, the headache, confusion, and dizziness often seen in the elderly with this condition can be easily confused with other conditions due to disease, the aging process, or medications (Collins & Stollerman, 1993; Dutt et al., 1992).

It is sometimes more difficult to elicit a clear history or problem description from elderly persons, particularly if they cannot communicate clearly because of a condition or medication. Thus, a degree of alertness is necessary in considering the presence of TB in an elderly individual, and the nurse needs to evaluate other risk factors such as living arrangements (in a nursing home or shelter) when deciding on further evaluation such as sputum smear, culture, and tuberculin skin testing.

Tuberculosis should be considered in the differential diagnosis when an elderly patient with multiple medical problems presents with an atypical respiratory illness. The testing and diagnostic procedures for the elderly person would be similar to that of persons of other ages. In considering tuberculin testing in the elderly, the nurse should be aware of the boosting phenomenon. This phenomenon occurs when there is enhancement of the pre-existing delayed hypersensitivity reaction from one tuberculin skin test to a subsequent one. Although it may appear that a conversion and new infection has taken place, it is a recall or booster rather than a conversion, and is most common in those over 55 years of age but diminishes in those older than 75 years (McDonald, 1993). Thus in the elderly a two-step procedure is recommended. If the first tuberculin skin test is nonreactive, then a second is done 1 to 2 weeks later. If the second is negative, then the person is classified as uninfected with TB. If it is positive, then it is considered the result of boosting (see Chapter 8) (McDonald, 1993; Yoshikawa, 1992).

Treatment

Just as in younger persons, TB should be treated in the elderly. The choice of the treatment plan for elderly persons should take into consideration

1. the possibility of adverse drug reaction to each anti-TB drug;
2. the potential for drug-drug interaction with other medications the elderly person is taking;
3. the presence of any serious underlying diseases; and
4. ability of the person to adhere to and carry out the therapy.

A description of drug regimens and plans to treat TB are given in Chapter 5. An important aspect of the treatment is assuring that the elderly person can take his or her prescribed medication; thus the nurse should assess the elderly patient's vision, memory, and mental clarity. Treatment should be as simple as possible while maintaining adequacy. Elderly persons may benefit from treatment supervision by a nurse, home-health aide, or family member. If therapeutically sound, the administration of medication for TB can be done two or three times a week rather than daily. Careful assessment and elicitation about signs and symptoms of medication side effects should be done (Dutt et al., 1993).

Whether or not to initiate preventive therapy with isoniazid (INH) in an elderly tuberculin reactor is somewhat controversial because the risk of hepatitis due to INH increases with age (Miller, 1993). Others believe that with careful monitoring (at least monthly for liver function and signs and symptoms of hepatitis) the benefit still outweighs the risk, particularly because of the importance of preventing the spread of TB to others and other reasons (Geiter, 1993; McDonald, 1993). Preventive therapy is discussed in Chapter 5.

SUMMARY

Certain populations require additional concern in regard to TB. These include persons with HIV disease, persons with HIV-disease, women, children, and the elderly. TB in each group requires particular assessment, planning, prevention, and treatment to address specific needs.

REFERENCES

Abernathy, R.S., Jacobs, R.F., & Stead, W.W. (1991). Six-months isoniazid-rifampin treatment for pulmonary tuberculosis in children. *American Review of Respiratory Diseases, 144*, 1221–1222.

Agrons, G.A., Markowitz, R.I., & Kramer, S.S. (1993). Pulmonary tuberculosis in children. *Seminars in Roentgenology, XXVIII,* 158–172.

Ajayi, V. (1980). *A textbook of midwifery.* Tropical Nursing and Health Science Series. London: Macmillan.

American Thoracic Society. (1990). Diagnostic standards and classification of tuberculosis. *American Review of Respiratory Disease, 142,* 725–735.

American Thoracic Society. (1994). Treatment of tuberculosis and tuberculosis infection in adults and children. *American Journal of Respiratory and Critical Care Medicine, 149,* 1359–1374.

Atkins, J.N. (1982). Maternal plasma concentration of pyridoxal phosphate during pregnancy: Adequacy of vitamin B6 supplementation during isoniazid therapy. *American Review of Respiratory Diseases, 126,* 714–716.

Bacon, C.S. (1905). Pulmonary tuberculosis as an obstetrical complication. *Journal of the American Medical Association, 45,* 1067–1070. In Leavitt, J.W. (Ed.). (1986). *Brought to bed: Childbearing in America* (pp. 68–69). New York: Oxford University Press.

Bakshi, S. S., Alvarez, D., Hilfer, C. L., Sordillo, E. M., Grover, R., & Kairam, R. (1993). Tuberculosis in human immunodeficiency virus-infected children. *American Journal of Diseases of Children, 147,* 320–324.

Barnes, P.F. & Barrows, S.A. (1993). Tuberculosis in the 1990s. *Annals of Internal Medicine, 119,* 400–410.

Barnes, P. F., Le, H. Q., & Davidson, P. T. (1993). Tuberculosis in patients with HIV infection. *Medical Clinics of North America, 77(6),* 1369–1390.

Berkowitz, R., Custan, D., & Mochizuki, T. (1986). *Handbook for prescribing medications during pregnancy.* (2nd ed.). Boston: Little, Brown.

Bowes, W. (1987). Tuberculosis. In Queenan, J. & Hobbins, J., (Eds.). *Protocols for high-risk pregnancies* (pp. 223–226). Oradell,: Medical Economics Books.

Brudney, K. & Dobkin, J. (1991). Resurgent tuberculosis in New York City. *American Review of Respiratory Diseases, 144,* 745–749.

Burrow, G.N., & Ferris, T.F. (1988). *Medical complications during pregnancy.* (3rd ed.). Philadelphia: W.B. Saunders.

Cantwell, M. F. Shehab, Z. M., Costello, A. M., Sands, L., Green, W. F., Ewing, E. P., Jr., Valway, S. E., & Onorato, I. M. (1994). Brief report: Congenital tuberculosis. *New England Journal of Medicine, 330,* 1051–1054.

Centers for Disease Control (1990a). Screening for tuberculosis and tuberculous infection in high-risk populations. *Morbidity and Mortality Weekly Report, 39 (RR-8),* 1–7.

Centers for Disease Control (1990b). Prevention and control of tuberculosis in facilities providing long-term care to the elderly. Recommendations of the advisory committee for elimination of tuberculosis. *Morbidity and Mortality Weekly Report, 39* (RR-10), 7–13.

Center for Disease Control (1991). Purified protein derivative (PPD)-tuberculin anergy and HIV infection: Guidelines for anergy testing and management of anergic persons at risk of tuberculosis. *Morbidity and Mortality Weekly Report, 40 (RR-5),* 27–33.

Centers for Disease Control. (1992). National Action Plan to Combat Multidrug Resistant Tuberculosis. *Morbidity and Mortality Weekly Report, 41*(RR–11), 1–71.

Centers for Disease Control and Prevention. (1992a). 1993 revised classification system for HIV infection and expanded surveillance case definition for AIDS among adolescents and adults. *Morbidity and Mortality Weekly Report, 41(RR–17)*, 1–19.

Centers for Disease Control and Prevention (1993a). Initial therapy for tuberculosis in an era of multidrug resistances. *Morbidity and Mortality Weekly Report, 42*(RR–7), 1–8.

Centers for Disease Control and Prevention (1993b). Tuberculosis among pregnant women—New York City, 1985–1992. *Morbidity and Mortality Weekly Report, 42*(31), 605, 611–612.

Centers for Disease Control and Prevention (1993c). Tuberculosis morbidity—United States, 1992. *Morbidity and Mortality Weekly Report, 42*, 696, 703–704.

Centers for Disease Control and Prevention (1994a). *1992 tuberculosis statistics in the United States.* Atlanta, GA, U. S. Department of Health and Human Services.

Centers for Disease Control. (1994b). Guidelines for preventing the transmission of *Mycobacterium tuberculosis* in health-care facilities, 1994. *Morbidity and Mortality Weekly Report, 43*(RR-13), 1–133.

Chebotareva, T.V. (1990). Tuberculosis and maternity. *Problemy Tuberkuleza, 11*, 6–7.

Collins, M. M. & Stollerman, G. H. (1993). Disseminated tuberculosis: A presumptive diagnosis. *Hospital Practice, 28 (12)*, 63–79.

Committee on Infectious Diseases. (1994). Screening for tuberculosis in infants and children. *Pediatrics, 93*, 131–134.

Couser, J. I. Jr. & Glassroth, J. (1993). Tuberculosis. An epidemic in older adults. *Clinics in Chest Medicine, 14*(3), 491–499.

De Cock, K., Soro, B., Coulibaly, I., & Lucas, S. (1992). Tuberculosis and HIV-infection in sub-Saharan Africa. *Journal of the American Medical Association, 268*, 1581–1587.

DeHaan, B., & Benson, C. (1992). *Tuberculosis.* Unpublished monograph. Chicago: Rush Presbyterian St Luke's Medical Center.

DiFerdinando, G. T. Jr., Glassroth, J., Hecht, F. M., & Stover, D. E. (1993). TB and HIV: A deadly synergy. *Patient Care, 27(14)*, 92–114.

Dorken, E., Grzybowski, S., & Allen, E.A. (1987). Significance of the tuberculin test in the elderly. *Chest, 92*, 237–240.

Dowling, P.T. (1991). Return of tuberculosis: Screening and preventive therapy. *American Family Physician, 43*, 457–467.

Drucker, E., Alcabes, P., Bosworth, W., & Sckell, B. (1994). Childhood tuberculosis in the Bronx, New York. *Lancet, 343*, 1482–1485.

Durukan, T., Urman, B., Yarali, H., Arikan, U., & Beykal, O. (1990). An abdominal pregnancy 10 years after treatment for pelvic tuberculosis. *American Journal of Obstetrics and Gynecology, 163*, 594–595.

Dutt, A. K., & Stead, W. W.(1992). Tuberculosis. *Clinics in Geriatric Medicine, 8*(4), 761–775.

Dutt, A. K., & Stead, W. W. (1993). Tuberculosis in the elderly. *Medical Clinics of North America, 77*(6), 1353–1368

Engel, N.S. (1989). Multiple drug therapy for pediatric tuberculosis. *MCN, 14,* 169.

Feigin, R.D., & Cherry, J.D. (1992). *Textbook of pediatric infectious diseases* (Vol. 2) (3rd ed.). Philadelphia: Saunders.

Frieden, T., & Fujiwara, P. (1992). Tuberculosis treatment. New York City Department of Health, *City Health Information, 11* (3), November.

Geiter, L. J. (1993). Preventive therapy for tuberculosis. *Lung Biology in Health and Disease, 66,* 241–250.

Glassroth, J. (1993). Diagnosis of tuberculosis. *Lung Biology in Health and Disease, 66,* 149–165.

Hamadeh, M. & Glassroth, J. (1992). Tuberculosis and pregnancy. *Chest, 101,* 1114–1120.

Harris, J. (1993). The babies of Bedford. *New York Times Sunday Magazine,* March 28.

Herbst, A. L., Mishell, D. R., Jr., Stenchever, M. A. & Droegemueller, W. (1992). *Comprehensive gynecology.* St. Louis: Mosby Year Book.

Horsburgh, C.R., Jr., & Pozniak, A. (1993). Epidemiology of tuberculosis in the era of HIV. *AIDS, 7(suppl 1),* S109-S114.

Hostetter, M.K., Iverson, S., Thomas, W., McKenzie, D., Dole, K., & Johnson, D.E. (1991). Medical evaluation of internationally adopted children. *New England Journal of Medicine, 325,* 479–485.

Hussey, G., Chisholm, T., & Kibel, M. (1991). Miliary tuberculosis in children: A review of 94 cases. *Pediatric Infectious Disease Journal, 10,* 832–836.

Jacobs, R. F. & Eisenach, K. D. (1993). Childhood tuberculosis. *Advances in Pediatric Infectious Diseases, 8,* 23–51.

Jacobs, R. F. & Starke, J.R. (1993). Tuberculosis in children. *Medical Clinics of North America, 77*(6), 1335–1351.

Johnson, M.P., & Chaisson, R.E. (1993) Tuberculosis and HIV disease. In Volberding, PA, & Jacobson MA (Eds). *AIDS Clinical Review 1993,* New York, Marcel Dekker, Inc., pp. 73–93.

Khouri, Y.F., Mastrucci, M.T., Hutto, C., Mitchell, C.D., & Scott, G.B. (1992). *Mycobacterium tuberculosis* in children with human immunodeficiency virus type 1 infection. *Pediatric Infectious Diseases Journal, 11,* 950–955.

Kurth, A. (1993). Reproductive issues, pregnancy and childbearing in HIV-positive women. In F.L. Cohen and J. D. Durham (Eds). *Women, Children and HIV/AIDS* (pp. 104–133). New York: Springer.

Lanphear, B.P., & Snider, D.E. (1991). Myths of tuberculosis. *Journal of Occupational Medicine, 33,* 501–504.

Lyon, L., Thomas, P. A., Caldwell, B., Admassur, E. (1992). Pediatric Spectrum of Disease Clinical Consortium. Tuberculosis in children born HIV-infected to mothers in New York City. Poster presented at the Eighth

International Conference on AIDS, July 19–24, 1992; PoB3649, Amsterdam, The Netherlands.

Maeur, M. (1992). Americans behind bars: A comparison of international rates of incarceration. New York: The Sentencing Project. In Machon, S. Prisoners with HIV/AIDS and TB/MDR-TB: The epidemic within the epidemic. Paper presented at the Eighth International Conference on AIDS, Amsterdam, July.

Margono, F., Mroueh, J., Garely, A., White, D., Duerr, A., & Minkoff, H. L. (1994). Resurgence of active tuberculosis among pregnant women. *Obstetrics & Gynecology, 83*, 911–914.

Mays, M. (1993). Tuberculosis. A comprehensive review for the certified nurse-midwife. *Journal of Nurse Midwifery, 38*(3), 132–139.

McDonald, R. J. (1993). Tuberculosis in the elderly. *Lung Biology in Health and Disease, 66*, 413–432.

McIntosh, E. D. G., Isaacs, D., Oates, R. K., Ryan, M. D., Mansour, A., & Falk, M. C. (1993). Extrapulmonary tuberculosis in children. *The Medical Journal of Australia, 158*, 735–740.

Merson, M. (1992). The current global situation of the HIV/AIDS pandemic. WHO: Global Programme on AIDS. Presented at the Eighth International Conference on AIDS. Amsterdam, July.

Miller, B. (1993). Preventive therapy for tuberculosis. *Medical Clinics of North America, 77*(6), 1263–1275.

Miller, F.J.W., & Thompson, M.D. (1992). Decline and fall of the tubercle bacillus: The Newcastle story 1882–1988. *Archives of Diseases in Children, 67*, 251–255.

Moulding, T. (1994). Pathophysiology and immunology: Clinical aspects. In D. Schlossberg (Ed). *Tuberculosis* (3rd ed), (pp. 41–50), New York: Springer-Verlag.

Mudido, P., & Speck, W. T. (1994). Perinatal tuberculosis. In D. Schlossberg (Ed). *Tuberculosis* (3rd ed), (pp. 277–279), New York: Springer-Verlag.

Narain, J.P., Raviglione, M.C., & Kochi, A. (1992). *HIV-associated tuberculosis in developing countries: Epidemiology and strategies for prevention.* Geneva: World Health Organization (WHO), 234–256.

Nemir, R.L. (1986). Perspectives in adolescent tuberculosis: Three decades of experience. *Pediatrics, 78*, 399–405.

Nemir, R.L., & Krasinski, K. (1988). Tuberculosis in children and adolescents in the 1980s. *Pediatric Infectious Disease Journal, 7*, 375–379.

Nemir, R. L., & O'Hare, D. (1991). Tuberculosis in children 10 years of age and younger: Three decades of experience during the chemotherapeutic era. *Pediatrics, 88*, 236–241.

Oberg, C.N. (1991). Tuberculosis in infancy: A case report. *Clinical Pediatrics, 30* (8), 498–501.

Pitchenik, A. E., & Fertel, D. (1992). Mycobacterial disease in patients with HIV infection. In G. P. Wormser (Ed.). *AIDS and other manifestations of HIV infection* (2nd ed., pp. 277–313), New York, Raven Press, Ltd.

Pritchard, J.A., MacDonald, P.C., & Gant, N.F. (1985). *Williams obstetrics.* (17th ed.). Norwalk: Appleton-Century-Croft.

Richardson, V., Zickler, C.F., & Wheat, L.J. (1991). Tuberculosis screening and treatment in children. *Journal of Pediatric Health Care, 5* (1), 11–17.

Rosenfeld, E.A., Hageman, J.R., & Yogev, R. (1993). Tuberculosis in infancy in the 1990s. *Pediatric Clinics of North America, 40(5),* 1087–1103.

Schluger, N. W., & Rom, W. N. (1994). Current approaches to the diagnosis of active pulmonary tuberculosis. *American Journal of Respiratory and Critical Care Medicine, 149,* 264–267.

Schutze, G.E., Rice, T.D., & Starke, J.R. (1993). Routine tuberculin screening of children during hospitalization. *Pediatric Infectious Disease Journal, 12* (1), 29–32.

Small, P. M. & Jacobson, M. A. (1994). Human immunodeficiency virus and mycobacterial infections. In D. Schlossberg (Ed). *Tuberculosis* (3rd ed), (pp. 265–275), New York: Springer-Verlag.

Smith, M. H. D. (1989). Tuberculosis in children and adolescents. *Clinics in Chest Medicine, 10,* 381–395.

Snider, D. (1984). Pregnancy and tuberculosis. *Chest, 86,* Supplement 10S – 13S.

Snider, D. & Hutton, M. (1989.) *Improving patient compliance in tuberculosis treatment programs.* Atlanta: CDC.

Snider, D., Layde, P., Johnson, M., and Lyle, M. (1980). Treatment of tuberculosis in pregnancy. *American Review of Respiratory Disease, 122,* 65–79.

Snider, D.E., Rieder, H.L., Combs, D., Bloch, A.B., Hayden, C.H., & Smith, M.H.D. (1988). Tuberculosis in children. *Pediatric Infectious Disease Journal, 7* (4), 271–278.

Starke, J.R. (1988). Modern approach to the diagnosis and treatment of tuberculosis in children. *Pediatric Clinics of North America, 35* (3), 441–464.

Starke, J. R. (1993). Tuberculosis in children. *Lung Biology in Health and Disease, 66,* 329–367.

Starke, J.R., & Kym, T.T. (1989). Tuberculosis in the pediatric population of Houston, Texas. *Pediatrics, 84,* 28–35.

Stead, W.W. (1981). Tuberculosis among elderly persons: An outbreak in a nursing home. *Annals of Internal Medicine, 94,* 606–610.

Stead, W.W., & Dutt, A.K. (1991). Tuberculosis in the elderly persons. *Annual Review of Medicine, 42,* 267–276.

Stead, W.W., & To, T. (1987). The significance of the tuberculin skin test in elderly persons. *Annals of Internal Medicine, 107,* 837–842.

Sweet, A. & Brown, E. (1991). *Fetal and neonatal effects of maternal disease.* St. Louis: Mosby Year Book, 139–144.

Use of BCG vaccines in the control of tuberculosis: A joint statement by the ACIP and the Advisory Committee for Elimination of Tuberculosis. (1988). *Morbidity and Mortality Weekly Report, 37*(43), 663–664.

Vallejo, J.G., & Starke, J.R. (1992). Tuberculosis and pregnancy. *Clinics In Chest Medicine, 13* (4), 693–707.

Warner, T.T., Khoo, S.H., & Wilkins, E.G. (1992). Reactivation of tuberculous lymphadenitis during pregnancy. *Journal of Infection, 24* (2), 181–184.

Weiss, G. (1991). The death of Charlotte Brönte. *Obstetrics & Gynecology*, *78*, 705–708.

Weltman, A. & Rose, D. (1993). The safety of Bacille Calmette-Guérin vaccination in HIV infection and AIDS. *AIDS*, *7*, 149–157.

Witter, F. (1988). Treatment of tuberculosis in pregnancy. In Niebyl, J. (Ed.). *Drug use in pregnancy* (pp. 37–43). Philadelphia: Lea & Febiger.

Wolinsky, E. (1992). Tuberculosis. In J.B. Wyngaarden, L.H. Smith, Jr., J.C. Bennett (Eds.). *Cecil Textbook of Medicine: Vol. 2.* (pp 1733–1745). Philadelphia:W.B. Saunders.

Wynn, R.M. (1988). *Obstetrics and gynecology: The clinical core* (pp. 216–217). Philadelphia: Lea & Febiger.

Yoshikawa, T. T. (1992). Tuberculosis in aging adults. *Journal of the American Geriatric Society*, *40*, 178–187.

12

TUBERCULOSIS AMONG THE HOMELESS: THE PINE STREET INN EXPERIENCE

Barbara McGinnis

THE HOMELESS

The homeless are men, women, and children without a permanent place to call home. Their usual "homes" include the streets, cars, subways, empty buildings, night shelters, soup kitchens, or day shelters. The homeless are persons who do not have customary and regular access to a conventional dwelling or residence (Rossi, Wright, Fisher, & Willis, 1987). It is difficult to estimate the number of homeless persons in the United States, but numbers range from 250,000 to 3 million. Demographic categories overlap. Homeless women (virtually unknown until about 20 years ago) account for about 25%, children under 18 years of age for about 15%, chronic substance abusers for about 33%, persons over 65 years of age for about 4%, and those with mental illness for about 33% (Brickner, Scharer, & McAdam, 1993). The majority are still middle-aged men in inner city urban areas (Nolan, Elarth, Barr, Saeed & Risser, 1991). Members of minority groups are disproportionately represented among the homeless. It is estimated that 38% are African-American, 12% are Hispanic and 3% are Native American; the approximate proportions in the general U.S. population are 12%, 6.5%, and 0.6%, respectively (Brickner et al., 1993). Being homeless is a devastating experience for the individuals, who are vulnerable to whatever the day brings, including assault, victimization, rape, adverse weather, dirt, and abuse. Prolonged standing or sitting can lead to venous stasis, leg edema, and ulcers. In addition, they may live in constant fear of losing their possessions or being attacked. These circumstances, coupled with mental illness, alcohol use, substance abuse, and the behavior and circumstances of those around them, mean that physical conditions and illnesses are often ignored until they are severe.

SHELTERS

Shelters vary in their accommodations, but are congregate living quarters. Typically, persons staying in a shelter are provided with a bed, cot, or a safe space on the floor. Supper is served, and beds are accessible at 6:00 P.M. This may seem early, but wake-up time is usually 5:00 A.M. Showers are ordinarily required of those able to take them. Counselors watch for signs of lice and scabies and provide treatment for them. Breakfast is served before people leave the shelter for the day. There is endless waiting in lines by those in shelters, and severe overcrowding occurs during mealtime, especially in the winter months. A shelter offers a harbor from the streets where violence and inclement weather threaten people's safety. Although shelters are designed for safety, when large numbers of people are together, infectious diseases can spread more rapidly. For example, in some shelters, beds may be separated by only 1 to 2 feet (Nolan, et al., 1991; Paul, et al., 1993). The association between crowding, poverty and tuberculosis has been recognized for decades. The Centers for Disease Control and Prevention (CDC) have made recommendations for ventilation within shelters recommending that it should be at or above 25 cubic feet of outside air per minute, per person. They also have recommended the use of supplemental upper room germicidal ultraviolet air disinfection to lessen transmission, and recommend that exposure at eye level be no greater than 0.2 microwatts per square centimeter over 8 hours (Centers for Disease Control, 1992) (see Chapter 9). Today, the crowding and poverty experienced by the

TABLE 12.1 Priorities for Tuberculosis Prevention and Control Activities Among Homeless Persons

- Detection, evaluation, and reporting of homeless persons who have current symptoms of active TB.
- Completion of an appropriate course of treatment by those diagnosed with active TB.
- Screening and preventive therapy for homeless persons who have, or are suspected of having, human immunodeficiency virus (HIV) infection.
- The examination and appropriate treatment of persons with recent TB that has been inadequately treated.
- Screening and appropriate treatment of persons exposed to an infectious case of TB. Because contacts are difficult to define in a shelter population, it is usually necessary to screen all residents of a shelter when an infectious case is identified.
- Screening and preventive therapy for homeless persons with known medical conditions that increase the risk of TB, e.g., diabetes mellitus.

Source: Centers for Disease Control (1992). Prevention and control of tuberculosis among homeless persons, *Morbidity and Mortality Report, 41* (RR-5), pg. 15.

homeless are compounded by immunosuppression due to malnutrition, drug abuse, and HIV-infection and by drug-resistant TB.

The risk of infection spread is heightened because the homeless often travel from shelter to shelter. The larger shelters in cities often have a health clinic or are visited by staff from public health agencies; however, the availability of even minimal health care services for the homeless varies greatly at shelters across the nation.

The large numbers of people in shelters can frighten and threaten homeless, mentally ill people who may choose instead to live on the street in self-imposed isolation; moreover, people with substance abuse problems and mental illness are frequently barred from shelters when their behavior is unmanageable for the shelter staff or threatens the safety of the other shelter residents. Living in alleys and under expressway bridges has become commonplace for the homeless. Under such conditions, the homeless receive very little food, health problems become worse, and many are the victims of crime.

When a person is living in an alley and is isolated from others, however, there is little risk of their exposure to TB. "Street people" often suffer from malnutrition and are more susceptible to a host of other diseases and conditions; thus, when they enter a shelter, they become the most susceptible to whatever contagious disease is current in residents of the shelter. Knowing these risks, many of the homeless, particularly the mentally ill, try to avoid shelters.

TUBERCULOSIS AND THE HOMELESS

Varying estimates have been made of the prevalence of TB among the homeless. In a recent study of a men's shelter in New York City, of the 134 residents participating, 79% had either past or present tuberculous infection (Paul et al., 1993). In another New York City men's shelter involving a total of 1,853 men, the overall rate of tuberculous infection was 42.8% including 6.0% with active tuberculosis (McAdam, Brickner, Scharer, Crocco, & Duff, 1990). In New York City, it has been estimated that there may be 600 to 1,000 homeless persons with active TB (Imperato, 1992). Nationally, the CDC estimate the prevalence of clinically active TB as ranging from 1.6% to 6.8% and the prevalence of tuberculous infection as 18% to 51% among the homeless (Centers for Disease Control, 1992).

A major problem is nonadherence or failure to complete TB treatment. Among one group of inner city patients in New York, including 68% who were homeless or in unstable housing, 89% failed to complete treatment, and homelessness was significantly associated with nonadherence (Brudney & Dobkin, 1991). The CDC have recommended that screening among the homeless consist of a chest radiograph and perhaps a sputum smear because results can be obtained quickly. Tuberculin skin testing can be done where the group is stable and can be located for reading of the test and completion of evaluation (Centers for Disease Control, 1987). Priorities for TB prevention and control among homeless persons are given in Table 12.1.

TUBERCULOSIS IN BOSTON AND THE PINE STREET INN

Tuberculosis has always been prevalent among homeless people in Boston. In 1971, for example, 41 of Boston's 299 cases of active TB were identified at the 240-bed Pine Street Inn, which is a shelter for homeless men and women in Boston. Because of this high number of cases, funding was allocated by the Massachusetts Department of Public Health TB Control for a TB Program on-site at the shelter. In May 1973, a full-time public health nurse began working at Pine Street Inn where that role was defined to include relating to the guests of the Inn as a friend rather than as a representative of the establishment. In 1974, of the 220 Boston cases of active TB only 18 were from Pine Street Inn, and in 1978, of the 270 Boston cases, 5 were from Pine Street Inn.

This important role dimension continues today at Pine Street Inn.

Having the nurse at the shelter daily allows for coordination of the TB Program, with evaluation and monitoring of surveillance and containment activities throughout the facility and liaison to the Inn's nursing clinic and other shelter staff, along with supervision of medications. The Pine Street Inn has an outreach van that visits street people daily from 9:00 P.M. until 5:00 A.M. The staff of this outreach van deliver food, clothes, and friendship to the homeless. They also provide transportation when needed or requested. An important part of the Inn's TB Program is education for staff and guests. A part-time physician has a weekly session to read chest radiographs, provide medical consultation, diagnose and prescribe treatment, and collaborate with the TB nurse who is responsible for the follow-up and referrals. Chest radiographs are available on-site twice each week.

In the early years of this shelter-based TB Program, the focus was on case finding and treatment of new cases of TB. In 1980, the number of shelter beds increased to 350 to meet the growing number of newly homeless people. Still the Inn became overcrowded, and more and more people shared the same air. On winter nights, as many as 300–400 people might sleep on the floors after the 350 beds were filled up. Resources were limited, forcing Inn staff to turn people away. Many homeless people were forced to be on the street where they became sicker and sicker. The Inn functioned as the city's only shelter until the mid-1880s, when the city and state opened up shelter programs to relieve overcrowding.

By 1993 Pine Street Inn was serving 640 homeless men and women. A nurses' clinic, in operation daily, is separate from the TB program. Clients are referred to the TB Program by local hospitals, detoxification facilities, staff from the Pine Street Inn's nurses' clinics and by counseling staff, and clinicians from Boston Health Care for the Homeless (BHCHP). Self-referrals are also accepted.

The Pine Street Inn TB Clinic

An outpatient TB clinic is offered at Pine Street Inn weekly. It provides diagnostic and treatment services to persons at risk for and with TB disease and infection. The goal is to interrupt progression and transmission of tuberculosis and to prevent tuberculous infection from progressing to disease. The clinic's location, directly off a lobby where clients are waiting for a bed ticket or meal, is a unique feature. The time for clinic is 6:30 P.M., after supper has been served but before beds are claimed for the night.

The public health nurse provides continuity for the TB Clinic by coordinating the services necessary and ensuring those services to guests and staff in the shelter. Clients are educated about the signs and symptoms, treatment, and epidemiology of TB. Expert medical staff provide TB services as recommended by the Centers for Disease Control and Prevention (CDC) and the American Thoracic Society and approved by the Massachusetts Department of Public Health (MDPH), Division of Tuberculosis Control. Client adherence is enhanced by the work of outreach workers, who play a major role in case finding, locating people on the street, establishing positive relationships, and watching for abnormal reactions to medications.

Licensed staff and Massachusetts-licensed equipment are available on-site. Specimens are obtained by the physician or nurse and sent out for testing. The results from sputum samples, collected by the nurse and sent to Boston City Hospital or the state laboratory, are received in the mail or by computer printout. Prescriptions for anti-TB medications are sent to the Boston City Hospital Outpatient Pharmacy. Filled prescriptions are picked up by a Pine Street Inn driver and delivered to the TB clinic. Medications are either given to the client or delivered to the Pine Street Inn Nurses Clinic for administering directly observed therapy (DOT) (see Chapter 7 and 10). The Massachusetts Department of Public Health and Boston Department of Health and Hospitals pay for the program and medications.

Case Finding

Contacts of a new case of TB who has a positive sputum smear for acid-fast bacilli (AFB) are identified by looking at the numbers next to the bed where the person who is the index case slept, and then comparing it to a bed roster for name identification. Persons in the eight surrounding beds are considered close contacts (see Chapter 10 for contact tracing). These persons are advised to have a tuberculin skin test and chest radiograph. Every effort is made by the shelter staff, using incentives and rewards, to help guests participate in this screening. If a shelter resident identified as a close contact is symptomatic and refuses to be tested, he or she is asked to leave the shelter until willing to cooperate. Persons with symptoms of active TB are masked and sent to the hospital immediately for admission. A health department nurse (this is usually the TB Homeless Liaison Nurse) makes a hospital visit to begin the patient teaching, contact identification, and case management. A person with a high index of suspicion for active TB must have three negative AFB smears before returning to the shelter.

Nursing Case Management

In Boston, the TB case managers are public health nurses who are employed by the Boston Department of Health and Hospitals (in Boston this is the equivalent of the Board of Health (BOH)). Every person considered to be a TB suspect or active case of TB is assigned a TB case manager (CM). At the first meeting, time is spent by the nurse CM with the patient and family to develop a mutually trusting relationship. Comprehensive data are collected in the health history, including psychosocial and spiritual assessment, precipitating factors, levels of functioning, coping skills, and available support persons. Development of a care plan, identification of close contacts, activation of interventions, evaluation of outcomes, and collaboration with physicians are the basis of the case management. The nurse CM ordinarily informs the local hospital staff about the shelter and BOH rules and regulations governing TB treatment for homeless people.

Acute medical care for the patient who has a tentative or actual diagnosis of TB is provided in local hospitals. Discharge of TB patients is arranged through the hospital social service with the TB case manager. Placement in another facility is orchestrated by the CM in conjunction with the State Health Department. When guests are not adherent to their anti-TB medication regimen, arrangements are made for long- term care at the TB Treatment Unit (TTU) (See Chapter 13) located at the Lemuel Shattuck Hospital (Lemuel Shattuck Hospital TB Treatment unit Mission Statement, 1993). Here, a secure inpatient setting provides medical treatment for clients who do not adhere to outpatient drug therapy and who are deemed a "public menace." Persons admitted to the TTU may consent to voluntary admission or may be court committed. The TTU is managed as a "Therapeutic Milieu," which allows staff as well as clients to focus on the underlying personality, addiction, and psychiatric problems that have affected clients' ability to recover from their medical disease. (Some patients may go through detoxification before admission.) Patients may stay on this unit until therapy is completed, up to 18 months. Nurse CMs participate in discharge planning and visit clients at least bimonthly.

An individual with active TB is considered nonadherent when there is evidence that no medication is being taken. In Boston, the policy for homeless people is that they must have DOT, which is available at shelters, detoxification facilities, halfway houses, and other residences. It is also available at the BCH TB clinic 5 days a week.

The menace law, under Sections 94A through C, Chapter 111 of the General Laws of Massachusetts, allows a person to be removed from a domicile or the street and into a medical treatment facility if the person

TABLE 12.2 Cases of TB in Boston and Three Homeless Shelters in Boston

Active Cases of TB		Cases of TB in the Homeless			
Year	Boston	Boston	S1	S2	S3
1983	137	2	2	na*	na
1984	131	19	16	2	0
1985	154	19	19	0	0
1986	141	17	17	0	0
1987	126	11	10	1	0
1988	132	16	9	4	1
1989	142	27	15	4	1
1990	149	26	14	1	1
1991	141	14	8	1	0

Note: S1 = Pine Street Inn
         S2 = Long Island Shelter
         S3 = Shattuck Shelter

*na = Not Applicable

has verified TB and is unwilling or unable to accept the medically prescribed treatment (General Laws of Massachusetts Chapter 111, Section 94–C, 1956). The person must also pose a serious danger to the health of the local community. After the legal procedures are completed and adequate proof is provided, the person may be remanded to the TTU (This unit is described in more detail in Chapter 13). The TB nurse CM is usually the person to implement the paperwork needed to enforce this law and testify in court. Evidentiary procedures are not easily implemented because the rights of the client must be considered; however, the health and safety of the public are paramount. Many times the patient does not understand the necessity of forced hospitalization, requiring the case manager to spend many hours to rebuild a trusting relationship with the patient.

A Tuberculosis Outbreak Report from the Pine Street Inn

Four patients with known histories of tuberculous infection or tuberculosis in the past were the probable index cases for a new outbreak of drug-resistant TB at the Pine Street Inn. Two are described briefly below. In January 1983, J.W., a white male with severe mental illness, presented with cavitary tuberculosis. Sputum smears were AFB positive and culture positive with *M. tuberculosis* that was resistant to isoniazid and streptomycin. He was admitted to the hospital and treated for 8 months and then transferred to a chronic care facility. His history showed that he had a clinical case of TB in 1978 when his sputum was AFB smear and culture negative. At that time, he had been treated with isoniazid, streptomycin, and ethambutol; however, he had not fully adhered to his medication regimen at that time.

In December of 1983, D.T., a Native American male with advanced alcoholism, was diagnosed with cavitary tuberculosis. Sputum smears were AFB positive and culture positive with *M. tuberculosis* that was resistant to isoniazid and streptomycin. He was admitted to the hospital for 6 months of treatment and returned to the shelter to complete 18 months of supervised medications. He often showed up in an intoxicated state to take his medications.

Late in 1983, a large number of active cases of TB began to appear in homeless people, and 27 were drug resistant to isoniazid and streptomycin. Most (22) of these cases were epidemiologically associated and appeared at Pine Street Inn (see Table 12.2) (Nardell, McInnis, Thomas, & Weidhaas, 1986). In November 1984, extensive screening was undertaken in the three larger shelters during a period of 4 nights. Of the 750 people in shelters, 586 agreed to take part in the screening. Of the 465 guests who had chest x-rays, 24 had films that were suspicious for TB. Several persons were hospitalized for further tests, and four cases were confirmed. Mantoux skin tests were given to 362 persons, but only 187 people could subsequently be located for a reading. Forty-two had reactive tests; of this group 38 had a chest x-ray and none had active disease (Barry et al., 1986). Cooperation by the clients and guests with the TB staff for screening was excellent because of the support by shelter staff members and intensive nursing intervention.

A computer listing was generated and sent to each shelter nightly before the testing began. This served as the data base for the current TB master list printed quarterly. As each person was given a Mantoux test and *Candida*, mumps, or tetanus skin tests as controls for anergy (see Chapter 8), a data sheet was started and completed when the tests were read.

In Boston in 1993, the TB Program for the eight homeless shelters (1,687 beds) and 2-day programs for homeless people are modeled after the program set up at the Pine Street Inn but without a TB clinic on site. We have the TB master list, a comprehensive and confidential information system giving us a printout of the tuberculin skin test and chest x-ray status of the homeless people in the shelters. With the advent of an increase in cases of HIV-disease, we are finding creative ways to keep the number of TB cases down. Our newer programs are the Boston Area TB HIV Homeless Outreach (BATBHHO) team (described in the next section) and the incentive program for homeless people on preventive therapy for TB.

BOSTON AREA TB/HIV HOMELESS OUTREACH (BATBHHO)

The BATBHHO team consists of four public health nurses and three outreach worker/case managers (ORW/CM). All are employed by the Boston Department of Health and Hospitals and work in the Tuberculosis Program or Infectious Disease (ID) Program. The team members are

Nurse 1:   Board of Health Liaison Nurse for Shelters and TB Clinic
Nurse 2:   Board of Health Nurse Stationed at a Local Shelter
Nurse 3:   TB Research and HIV/Infectious Disease Clinic Nurse
Nurse 4:   TB Research and HIV/Infectious Disease Clinic Nurse
ORW 1   TB Educator and Coordinator in Methadone Clinic
ORW/CM 2: Manager of Incentive Program
ORW/CM 3: Manager of Incentive Program and Infectious Disease Clinic ORW

This group is culturally and linguistically diverse. Weekly meetings are held to collaborate on strategies to increase the clients' adherence to the medical regimen. Staff meet regularly to discuss care issues and concerns of assigned clients. Clients are considered consumers for whom the best possible care is provided. When a group of high-risk individuals who need TB screening is identified, the team divides up the tasks and carries out the screening and follow-up. Client referrals are given to each member as needed, and time is focused on mutual support (BCH Incentive Program).

TB PREVENTIVE THERAPY INCENTIVE PROGRAM FOR THE HOMELESS

It has long been known that people who are have reactive tuberculin skin tests without symptoms find it difficult to continue to take preventive medication or keep clinic appointments. Incentives represent one small way to reward people for having interest in their health. To receive something tangible for taking care of oneself is not a subtle message.

The incentive program was designed and implemented to deliver preventive medication (DOT) to homeless persons at high risk of having tuberculous infection progress to active tuberculosis. This program is integrated with existing Health Department and Boston City Hospital (BCH) and homeless programs. In the future, the usefulness of the program will be evaluated by comparing adherence rates between this group and a group not offered incentives.

The staff have observed that coupons to a local restaurant and vouchers to be turned in for cash are the most effective incentives. Cash was selected as an incentive because local stores were unwilling to do business with the program. Although the stores did not say it directly, the owners/managers alluded to the idea that they did not want additional "poor" people shopping in their stores. Enablers and incentives are discussed in Chapter 7.

Two outreach workers are the case managers (ORWCM) for the incentive program. Each client, patient or guest participating in the program receives a weekly cash incentive for successfully taking medication in DOT. The cash cost for the program for each client is between $180 and $335 for 6 to 12 months of participation. These costs are less than 1 day of inpatient hospitalization for active TB. Arrangements for DOT are made by the case manager (ORWCM). On a weekly basis, the ORWCM checks with the persons observing the patient taking medication to verify adherence. The ORWCM meets the patient at a location previously agreed upon, and the voucher is issued and signed by the patient. This voucher can then serve like a traveler's check to be taken to a BCH cashier and signed again by the client. A signature matching the first one is all that is needed for identification to cash the voucher. This system was decided upon because many homeless people do not have the usual forms of identification.

The CM enters all transactions in the patient's record for the program. Current addresses, phone numbers the network of support persons, strategies that worked or did not work, where and when visits were made, all become part of this record. When the therapy is completed, the record is filed to be evaluated in the future.

The case manager is usually an outreach worker. Each time the patient and ORWCM meet, the client is reminded that he or she is participating in a program by caring for himself or herself. Teaching about various health concerns is integrated into casual conversation. The ORWCM becomes an advocate for the patient when needed. This caring relationship for the patient is often the first time a homeless person has established a bond with another person in many years. Another valuable aspect of the program is that patients will say they have not previously completed any project and to do so makes them feel proud. The homeless men and women who are the center of the TB programs form a rich and diverse community with special needs. We believe that it is important to provide culture-specific nursing care. The staff believe that the client, patient or guest should direct the care they receive. Acceptance of this view means that a primary staff role is to design appropriate programs to meet client needs. If success in public health nursing is measured in outcomes, the staff have learned to adjust outcomes on a daily basis. In caring for homeless people, staff collaborate to make Boston safe and healthy for all.

Based upon the experience of this author, preventive therapy for TB can be successfully delivered to a mobile, homeless population through a case management program that offers DOT and incentives. Continued surveillance will identify the essential elements of this approach in decreasing TB morbidity in this high risk population.

REFERENCES

Barry, M.A., Wall, C., Shirley, L.,Bernardo, J., Schwingl, P., Brigandi, E. & Lamb, G. A. (1986). Tuberculosis screening in Boston's homeless shelters. *Public Health Report, 101*, 487–494.

Brickner, P. W., Scharer, L. L., & McAdam, J. M. (1993). Tuberculosis in homeless populations. *Lung Biology in Health and Disease, 66*, 433–454.

Brudney, K. & Dobkin, J. (1991). Resurgent tuberculosis in New York City. *American Review of Respiratory Disease, 144*, 745–749.

Centers for Disease Control (1987). Tuberculosis control among homeless populations. *Morbidity and Mortality Weekly Report, 36*, 257–260.

Centers for Disease Control (1992). Prevention and control of tuberculosis among homeless persons. *Morbidity and Mortality Weekly Report, 41(RR-5)*, 13–23.

General Laws of Massachusetts Chapter 111, Section 94 A–C. 1956.

Imperato, P. J. (1992). Tuberculosis, AIDS and homelessness. *Journal of Community Health, 17*, 187–189.

McAdam, J. M., Brickner,P. W., Scharer, L. L., Crocco, J. A. & Duff, A. E. (1990). The spectrum of tuberculosis in a New York City men's shelter clinic (1982–1988). *Chest, 97*, 798–805.

Nardell, E., McInnis, B., Thomas, B., & Weidhaas, S. (1986). Exogenous reinfection with tuberculosis in a shelter for the homeless. *New England Journal of Medicine, 315*, 1570–1575.

Nolan, C. M., Elarth, A. M., Barr, H., Saeed, A. M., & Risser, D. R. (1991). An outbreak of tuberculosis in a shelter for homeless men. *American Review of Respiratory Disease, 143*, 257–261.

Paul, E. A., Lebowitz, S. M., Moore, R. E., Hoven, C. W., Bennett, B. A., & Chen, A. (1933). Nemesis revisited: tuberculosis infection in a New York City men's shelter. *American Journal of Public Health, 83*, 1743–1745.

Rossi, P.H., Wright, J.D., Fisher, G.A., Willis, G. (1987). The urban homeless: estimating composition and size. *Science, 235*, 1336–1341.

13

LONG-TERM INPATIENT CARE FOR TUBERCULOSIS: A TREATMENT OF LAST RESORT

Linda Singleton and Maria A. Tricarico

Today long-term care (LTC) for active tuberculosis (TB) is needed only when outpatient treatment either does not succeed, despite all efforts, or the medical complexity is such that treatment is best managed in the hospital setting. Typically, LTC is a last resort measure for those who will not adhere to therapy. However, medical complexity reasons for admission are on the increase. Although most medical admissions usually require shorter stays, a new profile is emerging in the current TB epidemic of patients with medical management problems coexisting with nonadherence, multidrug-resistant disease, a chemotherapy regime with many adverse effects, and at times coinfection with HIV disease.

Other chapters in this book review community responsibilities for tuberculosis control, as well as methodologies to enhance patient adherence to treatment. This chapter explores the need for long-term inpatient care, the changing patient profile, ethical responsibilities, admission and discharge planning, and recommendations for holistic and comprehensive care.

BACKGROUND

Historical Perspective

When the old-fashioned TB sanitoriums in the United States closed by the late 1960s and early 1970s, outpatient services were expected to successfully manage uncomplicated cases of active tuberculosis. Some patients with special problems continued to require periods of hospitalization for reasons of nonadherence and medical management. However, a positive sputum culture alone was no longer a reason for hospital admission.

Historically, the older, nonadherent male alcoholic is an example of a person who continued to be admitted to hospitals because of remaining uncooperative about to therapy despite all efforts. In an effort to address some of the issues related to caring for the alcoholic tuberculosis patient, the American Thoracic Society issued an official policy statement in 1977 outlining some strategies for successful outpatient treatment. At that time the value of hospitalization for the totally uncooperative patient was still debatable and the report stated that "A satisfactory modality of management remains to be developed." (American Thoracic Society, 1977, p.560).

The policy of eliminating all long-term beds continues to be debated by TB control practitioners and managers. In 1986, Yeager and Medinger took issue with this policy and stated that "every city or state in the United States would profit from maintaining a handful of these beds for a small number of patients who have tuberculosis" (p. 752). They cited the homeless and those who require retreatment due to partial or total nonadherence with recommended therapy as the individuals who would need long-term care (Yeager & Medinger, 1986). In response to this article, Sbarbaro and Iseman (1986) agreed that there may be a need for long-term care facilities but emphasized the importance of community-based, directly observed therapy (DOT) programs before resorting to institutions. In New York City, where TB cases have steadily increased since 1979, Brudney and Dobkin (1991) described the reasons why the system of control failed. In 1978 nearly all of the 1,000 designated TB beds were eliminated from the New York City budget and the allocations for outpatient care were severely reduced as well, leaving insufficient resources for all levels of TB control. In addition to aggressive community-based supervision, Brudney et al. recommended prolonged initial hospitalization and residential TB treatment facilities for the homeless and the nonadherent.

In an effort to learn more about the inpatient facilities utilized by others for TB control throughout the country, in 1988 the Massachusetts Department of Public Health, (MDPH) Division of Tuberculosis Control, conducted a survey of state, territorial, and big city health departments. Forty-six percent of the respondents answered "yes" to the question, "Do you operate or contract for inpatient intermediate or long-term care services for patients who cannot be managed as outpatients?" In response to questions regarding the type of facility used, 77% used acute care hospitals, 35% used chronic care hospitals, 23% used more than one type of hospital, and 30% said they used other types of facilities. The "other types" included nursing homes; residential living centers; correction houses; state and county hospitals, including mental health; and boarding homes. One state still owned and operated a TB sanitorium (Singleton et al., 1989).

Clearly, based on this survey, practitioners of TB control continue to find it necessary to treat some individuals with long-term inpatient care. As indicated below, the optimal type of facility is still subject to debate among TB controllers.

Types of Facilities

Quite correctly, practitioners have argued that utilizing acute care hospitals to treat patients for nonadherence can be quite expensive and ineffective without special provisions and coordinated efforts from state and local health departments. Hospitals today are concerned with cost containment and subject to Diagnosis Related Group (DRG) reimbursement schedules (Yeager & Medinger, 1986). Early discharges based on utilization review may be appropriate for the hospitals but inappropriate for the patient who has a long history of nonadherence with community-based treatment. However, acute care beds may be appropriate for the treatment of those with complicated drug-resistant disease. Second-line drugs may have more adverse side effects, may be poorly tolerated, and require frequent monitoring and specialized medical expertise. (Sbarbaro et al., 1986) (see Chapter 5). The use of boarding or living facilities were also recommended for TB patients unable to remain in a community long enough to complete treatment. Such individuals might lack family and social support, have mental illnesses, and be chronically unemployed (Sbarbaro et al., 1986). The option of low-cost residential settings is an attractive one to most communities; however, they are only cost effective if the patients are motivated to remain in one place throughout their therapy.

To alleviate some of the problems associated with caring for the homeless TB patients, New York City established a special shelter unit in a large city shelter to house approximately 80 homeless men diagnosed with TB. This shelter is a positive incentive to continue with DOT because it gives the men a designated bed in an uncrowded environment for the duration of their therapy. If they leave the shelter for longer than the allowed time or if they refuse to keep the general rules, they lose their bed. Unfortunately, some individuals cannot maintain this lifestyle and they do not complete therapy under these conditions.

The Massachusetts Department of Public Health, Division of Tuberculosis Control, also explored the use of a shelter for treating some patients. The Division contracted for three beds in a state run shelter with a medical respite unit. The patients with an acid-fast bacilli (AFB) sputum smear-negative active TB would be guaranteed a bed and were not required to leave the shelter during the day. In addition, the shelter offered an attractive case management plan that included special services such as social services, addictions treatment, and medical management. The shelter guest with TB only needed to take his or her medication as prescribed and follow the general shelter rules. Unfortunately, this low cost alternative to more expensive beds was underutilized because many patients in need of long-term care were not considered reliable enough to remain under the limited supervision of the shelter. Several shelter guests, in fact, left for the street and other alternative lifestyles before completing therapy (Etkind, Boutotte, Ford, Singleton, & Nardell 1991).

As described in Chapter 11, the Massachusetts Department of Public Health, Division of Tuberculosis Control, has also maintained a single "Tuberculosis Treatment Unit" (TTU) since 1970 when the last sanitorium was converted to a chronic care hospital. This TTU has been necessary for the care of patients who did not complete outpatient therapy and needed a more structured environment in order to complete treatment. Further description of the use of this unit, and how the care changed to meet the needs of the population, will be discussed in more detail in the remainder of this chapter.

Although the facilities utilized during the first half of this century no longer exist, some experts believe that a regional or national "sanitorium-type" facility would be useful for people with multidrug-resistant

TB with complex problems who remain AFB sputum smear-positive. Such individuals are considered a continuous threat to society and cannot be placed in most facilities. This kind of facility, supported by federal tax dollars, would provide an environment suitable to residential living but with the necessary medical and nursing support (Sbarbaro et al., 1986). Questions concerning the need for long-term beds continue to be asked, but most practitioners agree that such alternative facilities should be available for those who cannot be managed successfully as outpatients and ultimately become treatment failures.

THE NEED FOR A NEW MODEL OF CARE

The Changing Patient Profile

The profile of persons requiring inpatient long-term care (LTC) continues to change with the social and economic conditions prevalent in the society. As expected, the same persons who are the most difficult to treat as outpatients are at the greatest risk for not completing successful therapy and for needing inpatient care. In Massachusetts, Etkind et al. (1991) identified a group of "hard to treat" patients as those who were "not cured by 6 to 12 months of chemotherapy—usually because of incomplete or erratic treatment leading to drug resistance" (p. 275). Attributable causes of the incomplete or erratic treatment included inappropriate medical care, financial and cultural barriers, mental illness, homelessness, and substance abuse (Etkind et al., 1991).

Drug-resistant TB in the hard-to-treat population carries its own cost with repeat acute care hospitalizations, prolonged and often toxic treatment regimes, increased community nursing time, and the risk of infecting or causing disease in others. During an outbreak of isoniazid (INH) and streptomycin- resistant tuberculosis among the homeless, Massachusetts found that long-term care was the most effective method for controlling the spread of the disease to others. The index case initially presented with drug-sensitive disease in 1960 but developed drug-resistant disease by 1974 secondary to nonadherence. His disease reactivated again in 1983 at which time he infected many other guests in a homeless shelter and ultimately caused INH-and streptomycin-resistant disease in more than 60 other people (Nardell, McInnis, Thomas, Weidhaas , 1986). In order to control the outbreak, 40 of the cases required long-term care, averaging 97 days each, in a tuberculosis unit in a chronic care hospital (Weidhaas, Nardell, & Ford, 1988). Many of these patients were given repeat opportunities for outpatient care but were not successful in spite of all efforts. When others left against medical advice, significant resources were required in order to restart treatment.

As of November 1988, 75% of the INH and streptomycin-resistant homeless TB cases who were hospitalized finished treatment, as compared with 53% of hospitalized nonresistant cases. For homeless cases not hospitalized at all, 35% of the drug-resistant cases completed therapy compared to a 33% completion rate for nonresistant homeless cases (Etkind et al., 1991). Presumably, these costs could have been avoided if the index case received high priority treatment, including long-term care when outpatient treatment services failed.

It became apparent in the late 1980s that a new patient profile had emerged causing treatment difficulties for the TTU as well as the community. Nonadherence in the community was magnified by difficult-to-find "street" homeless and substance abusers whose social and economic problems were all encompassing and for whom treatment for TB was a low priority. Medical problems common to this population created more case management issues. The TTU, once accustomed to a relatively peaceful environment, now faced more challenges than ever before. There were episodes of uncontrolled abusive and violent behaviors, patients leaving against medical advice, evidence of contraband, and complicating illnesses brought on by coinfection with human immunodeficiency virus (HIV) infection. In a prospective study of 224 TB patients admitted to a large public hospital in New York City, Brudney et al. (1991) were able to track the adherence and completion rates of 178 of these patients who were discharged on tuberculosis treatment. Nonadherence was significantly associated with homelessness, alcoholism, and the absence of symptomatic HIV disease. Females were somewhat less adherent than were males, and crack users were totally nonadherent.

Another change in the patient profile is demonstrated by the recent rise in drug-resistant tuberculosis in the United States. It is a serious concern for public health as well as tuberculosis control practitioners. An increasing proportion of the cases occur among the homeless, those with substance abuse problems or mental illness, foreign-born persons, and groups with difficult socioeconomic problems that lead to nonadherence with TB treatment (Centers for Disease Control and Prevention, 1992). Since drug resistance is easily developed in the nonadherent patient who perhaps takes some but not all of the drugs or takes them intermittently over a period of time (see Chapter 5), it is extremely important to utilize all necessary measures to prevent this from occurring, especially in high-risk populations who are difficult to treat. It is not difficult to imagine problems encountered by community-based treatment programs trying to case manage homeless substance abusers who have drug-resistant TB and as well as HIV-disease.

The threat to the public health clearly emerged when multidrug-resistant tuberculosis (MDR-TB) spread quickly in several hospitals and prisons where vulnerable populations with HIV/AIDS disease shared the same breathing air. In an investigation of seven outbreaks of MDR-TB by the federal Centers For Disease Control and Prevention (CDC), from 1990 through early 1992, it was found that most patients were both TB and HIV- infected and that the mortality rate was very high, ranging from 72% to 89%. Health-care workers and prison guards were also at risk for tuberculous infection and tuberculosis (Centers for Disease Control and Prevention, 1992).

A New Model of Care

As noted earlier, The MDPH, Division of Tuberculosis Control, has maintained a TTU since 1970, in a chronic care hospital. As the patient profile changed, the challenges in operating the TTU increased. The operational demands of running a unit for older, male alcoholics gave way to the complexities of addressing the needs of younger, drug addicted, homeless, mentally ill, and possibly HIV-infected men and women. In 1990, the unit was relocated to a Department of Public Health hospital with acute care capability. The premise and conceptual framework for the unit was modified to include treatment and rehabilitation of concomitant medical and psychosocial problems as well as the tuberculosis. The hypothesis was that if the etiology of the nonadherence could be addressed, the chance of successful treatment would increase and the rate of recidivism would decrease.

To that end, the unit was developed as a medical-surgical unit operating within the context of a psychiatric therapeutic milieu. A therapeutic milieu is usually defined as a carefully arranged environment that allows the patient to understand the effect that his or her behavior has on other patients and staff. This understanding assists the patient in developing the social and emotional skills necessary to function in everyday life. On the new TTU, this skill development was seen as critical in altering the nonadherent behavior and allowing the patient to return to a less-restrictive treatment option such as DOT on an outpatient basis.

The milieu was structured within several critical parameters:
- All patients would be offered the option of voluntary admission. (Massachusetts has the legal ability to commit someone to a TTU as a "public menace");

- The unit would be locked;
- Patients would be able to earn off-unit and off-campus privileges based on their adherence with published unit rules;
- A schedule of activities and therapeutic groups, including psychotherapy would be offered;
- Addictive behaviors would be addressed on a 12-Step Program model;
- Unit issues would be addressed in a "Community Meeting" attended by staff and patients;
- Patients would participate in certain unit jobs like maintaining the community kitchen and watering plants;
- Patients, by virtue of the choices they made, would be in control of what happened to them; and
- The rights to self-determination, privacy, respect, and dignity would be carefully protected for everyone on the unit.

Upon admission, each patient would be carefully apprised of all these parameters and provided with written material for reference. Family and significant others would receive the same information as appropriate and according to the patient's wishes.

In this TTU, the care and treatment of each individual is assessed, planned, implemented, and evaluated by a multidisciplinary and multiagency team. Although many disciplines participate in patient care on the TTU, it is primarily nurse driven. The public health nurses in the field do the case management; the nurses in the TB Division of the Department of Public Health share case management to ensure a consistent, comprehensive approach; a psychiatric clinical nurse specialist and a psychiatric clinical social worker manage the milieu; a nurse manager and a clinical coordinator run the daily operations; and a nurse practitioner provides most of the medical care. A pulmonologist is the medical director of the unit. Physicians with expertise in infectious disease, internal medicine, surgery, radiology, and psychiatry are all consultants on the unit.

The TTU is regarded as the option of last resort. Patients must have a track record of failure in the community after attempting all reasonable measures to ensure adherence before he or she is a candidate for the unit. "Adherent" persons may also be admitted to the Unit. Such individuals include those whose medical care is best managed by the TTU staff and those who are infectious but cannot be isolated in such places as shelters or crowded, communal living facilities. Discharge planning begins on the day of admission. Comprehensive evaluation and care planning are accomplished in bimonthly multidisciplinary and multiagency meetings. Neither the hospital staff nor the field staff dominate. Decisions are based on what will best benefit both the patient and public health and, importantly, upon the patient's stated goals. At times, the patient's goal may be simply to get out of the unit. If it can be determined that there is a reasonable chance of successful treatment outside the unit, then the patient is prepared to go. This is difficult for the staff if none of the other issues are resolved. The primary goal of the unit is effective containment and treatment of difficult TB cases, so it must be the status of the TB treatment that drives admission and discharge. Staff members often deal with their very real disappointment that a patient may not wish to resolve his or her substance abuse or homelessness while on the TTU. If significant mental illness is diagnosed during admission, the court may be petitioned to determine competence, in which case treatment of the mental illness becomes a second determining factor in discharge planning.

The question must be asked, "Why pour resources into a comprehensive program, when all of the components do not directly address the primary objective of the project?" In response, one must recall that the original hypothesis stated that addressing the root of the nonadherence would increase the likelihood of successful treatment and reduce repeated attempts. The initial data collected over the first year of operation of the new TTU revealed that 14% of those discharged were readmitted in comparison with 30% readmitted in the prior program. The reasons for the difference are varied, and more data must be collected and analyzed to draw firm conclusions. These reasons may include 1) having a locked unit (and therefore fewer escapes); 2) including the patient as an active partner in the treatment planning and evaluation (thereby fostering a more cooperative, and therefore more adherent patient situation); 3) treating major mental illness; and 4) treating substance abuse.

An important factor in assessing the efficacy of the new TTU model is the level of medical and/or surgical care provided on the unit. Extensive pulmonary disease may be prevalent in a population of nonadherent TB patients, some of whom have MDR-TB. Respiratory therapy, chest tubes, parenteral chemotherapy, and perioperative and postoperative care are provided as required. HIV disease plays an increasingly significant role in the type of services necessary for this group. Again, parenteral chemotherapy, total parenteral nutrition, and a wide spectrum of medical and surgical procedures are delivered as the care demands. Treatment for sexually transmitted diseases, cancer, diabetes, and other chronic and terminal diseases has also been necessary. Service delivery for such a complex case mix within the facility of an acute care hospital is proving to be more efficient and cost effective than facility-to-facility transfers and fragmentation of treatment plans. Providing all the care within one organization also prevents the interruption of the psychosocial rehabilitation because it is the same multidisciplinary team that coordinates all the care.

It is critical to note that staffing levels and skill mix must be adequate to address the dual approach to patient care. Cross training staff in medical, surgical, and psychiatric nursing issues is essential to achieve the full benefit of the comprehensive service delivery model. Even with an adequate, well-trained staff, the unit is highly stressful leading, to staff burnout. Regular staff meetings and support groups conducted by a psychiatric clinical nurse specialist provide some relief for staff who must cope with angry, confused, frightened and sometimes violent people. At the same time that the nurse's approach must be consistent with a behavioral-psychiatric treatment plan, she or he must deliver skilled medical and surgical care, implement universal and respiratory precautions, and maintain an environment conducive to mental, physical, and spiritual healing. This all creates a very difficult work situation, setting the stage for the aforementioned stress and burnout. There is no easy answer to this problem. Ongoing staff feedback, with clinical and administrative support, allows the program to develop new methods for problem solving. Tuberculosis is an old threat that has evolved into a new challenge for the '90s. It is the evolution of treatment approaches that will produce the answers for weary staff and apprehensive patients.

PROTECTING INDIVIDUAL RIGHTS AND PUBLIC HEALTH

Practitioners in tuberculosis control are often in the position of balancing the interests of public health with the rights of individuals. Respect for other persons requires that individuals have the opportunity to be in charge of their own health care, including where they will or will not go for treatment. Limitations on individual liberties are allowed only when there is evidence that others will be harmed as a result of personal behaviors. It is necessary, therefore, to continuously assess and justify whose rights will take priority. Restricting individual rights is not an alternative to a failing public health infrastructure or a limited community-based TB program. Although it is not possible to immediately solve the problems that lead to nonadherence, such as homelessness and substance abuse, every effort must be made to maximize access to care and provide the necessary enablers and incentives. Long before inpatient care is considered for nonadherence, we must ask ourselves whether the patient is failing or whether the system is failing the patient. For example, the public health system fails when a patient, who does not have the resources to ride across town to keep a DOT appointment, is labeled "nonadherent." It is when the resources are provided and the patient agrees with the care plan, but refuses to follow through, that the practitioner needs to evaluate the harm imposed upon public health. An alternate plan such as a signed contract between the patient and the practitioner, outlining the possible consequences of not adhering to the care plan, may be all that is necessary to reach a mutual agreement. Such least restrictive measures are essential to the preservation for individual rights.

Many states have laws that allow them to involuntarily confine patients with tuberculosis. One court case that paved the way for this authority was *Jacobson v. Massachusetts*, in which it was ruled that "upon the principle of self-defense, of paramount necessity, a community has the right to protect itself against an epidemic of disease which threatens the safety of its members." (*Jacobson v. Massachusetts, 1904*). Although the legal mandates of each state will vary, it is incumbent upon the practitioner to document very carefully that a nonadherent patient is indeed a threat to public health and all least-restrictive measures have been employed prior to limiting freedom.

When the "last resort" measure of inpatient care seems inevitable, the patient should be offered the opportunity for voluntary admission before legal steps are taken. Thus he or she continues to be part of the care plan and can maintain an element of personal dignity. However, important to ultimate success is what happens to the individual who is released back to the community. As Felton and Ford (1993) put it, if that person returns to "homelessness, unemployment, and widespread drug abuse, tuberculosis in our inner cities is here to stay."(p. 498).

SUMMARY

Long-term inpatient care for the treatment of tuberculosis is still necessary for some patients who cannot be managed successfully in the outpatient setting. Long-term care should always augment a strong community-based public health infrastructure and never replace it. This chapter reviewed long-term care from the historical perspective and describes recent events that change the methods of treatment necessary in order to help patients complete therapy and, thereby, protect the public health. The new profile of patients who do not complete successful outpatient treatment demands a creative approach for an inpatient model that manages nonadherent behavior while treating for tuberculosis. This model must balance the interests of the public health with the rights of the individual. This is particularly important because many of the patients considered for institutionalization for treatment are poor and nonwhite

(Felton & Ford, 1993). Patients in long-term care settings should be treated with dignity and respect and remain part of a care plan that protects their health, as well as the health of the public. That plan must include what happens to the individual on discharge.

REFERENCES

American Thoracic Society (1977). Treatment of tuberculosis in alcoholic patients. *American Review of Respiratory Disease, 116*, 559–561.

Brudney K., & Dobkin J. (1991). Resurgent tuberculosis in New York City. *American Review of Respiratory Disease, 144*,745–749.

Centers for Disease Control and Prevention. (1992). National action plan to combat multidrug- resistant tuberculosis. *Morbidity and Mortality Weekly Report, 41(No RR-11)*, 1–48.

Etkind S., Boutotte, J., Ford, J., Singleton L., & Nardell, E. A. (1991). Treating hard to treat tuberculosis patients in Massachusetts. *Seminars in Respiratory Infections, 6*, 273–282.

Felton, C. P., & Ford, J. G. (1993). Tuberculosis in the inner city. *Lung Biology in Health and Disease, 66*, 483–503.

Jacobson v Massachusetts, 197 U.S. 11 (1904). In Annas, G. J. (1993). Control of tuberculosis—the law and the public's health. *New England Journal of Medicine, 328*, 585–588.

Nardell, E., McInnis, B., Thomas, B., & Weidhaas, S. (1986). Exogenous reinfection with tuberculosis in a shelter for the homeless. *New England Journal of Medicine, 315*, 1570–1575.

Sbarbaro J. A. & Iseman M.D. (1986). Baby needs a new pair of shoes. *Chest, 90*, 754–755.

Singleton, L., Weidhaas-Etkind, S., Nardell, E.A., & Hendricks K. (1989). Tuberculosis Services—Who Pays? Poster presented at the American Thoracic Society, International Conference, Cincinnati, OH, May, 1989.

Weidhaas S., Nardell E., & Ford J. (1988). The economic consequences of a single, uncontrolled case of drug resistant tuberculosis among the homeless. *American Review of Respiratory Disease, 137 (suppl)*, 23 (abstr).

Yeager H. Jr., & Medinger A. E. (1986). Tuberculosis long-term care beds: Have we thrown out the baby with the bathwater? *Chest, 90*, 752–754.

14

TUBERCULOSIS: AN OVERVIEW OF ETHICAL AND LEGAL ISSUES

Jerry D. Durham

Effective treatment for TB, introduced over the past 40 years, resulted in annual decreases in the number of TB cases until 1985. For most infected persons, cure was possible, provided they adhered to recommended chemotherapy. Funding, scientific advances, and new drug therapies suffered from a lack of interest on the part of those responsible for public health policy. For those few—mostly from marginalized groups—for whom cure was not possible, TB came to mean "too bad."

The causes of the resurgence of TB in this country were not unpredictable. Many of these causes, briefly summarized here, are not new: decreased surveillance and control of TB; lack of access to medical care; inattention to health care facility engineering; an increase in susceptible populations; the HIV and drug use epidemic; the increase in homelessness and poverty; increases in populations housed in congregate settings (e.g., prisons and nursing homes); and immigration of populations from nations with a high incidence of TB (Gostin, 1993). Much attention has recently been given to these causes, attended by considerable finger pointing. A renewed interest in TB, coupled with a realization of the archaic state of knowledge about the disease, has resulted in increased government funding to improve surveillance and control activities and research relative to TB since the late 1980s (Centers for Disease Control, 1990, a,b;1992; Office of Technology Assessment, 1993; U.S. Congress, 1992, 1993; U.S. Department of Health and Human Services, 1988).

OVERVIEW OF ETHICAL/LEGAL CONCERNS

The factors noted above, particularly when coupled with the HIV epidemic, have raised new concerns about how to control the spread of TB. Because persons with HIV are at greater risk for TB than the general population, some draconian measures suggested to contain the HIV epidemic have resurfaced in discussions about TB. Although the ways in which TB and HIV are spread are very different, fears about contagion have increased among Americans over the past decade as a result of the HIV epidemic, leading to growing concerns about the need to contain TB before it becomes a greater public health problem. Moreover, concerns about the morbidity and mortality associated with MDR-TB have led to the general understanding that the current TB epidemic is not "deja vu, all over again" (United Hospital Fund, 1992, p.vii).

Although the TB and HIV/AIDS epidemics are different in many ways, they are similar in that both "engage the often competing interests of personal liberty and public health and find in opposition the dictates of professional authority and the imperatives of institutional management" (United Hospital Fund, 1992, vii). In some ways, the TB epidemic may pose greater ethical and legal challenges to policy makers because, although HIV generally is spread through consensual behaviors, TB is spread through the air that others breathe. In other words, the organism that causes TB cannot be avoided through chosen behaviors; thus, because the person with active TB potentially poses a health risk to the general population, should not their individual liberties be restricted when their adherence to treatment is inadequate? The degree to which individual liberty of those with active TB should be restricted remains a primary challenge to public health authorities and civil libertarians. This concern is particularly difficult for those charged with protecting the public's health when individuals with active TB do not adhere to prescribed interventions. One approach—mandatory directly observed therapy (DOT)—has been suggested as a means to increase adherence to

TABLE 14.1 Recommendations of Working Group on TB and HIV. United Hospital Fund (1992)

1. Will effective TB Control Programs Necessitate Mandatory HIV Screening?
   A. Knowledge of an individual's HIV status is not necessary for an effective TB screening program; therefore, there is neither legal nor ethical justification for abrogating the legal requirement that individuals provide informed consent prior to HIV testing.
   B. There is no public health justification for unconsented, routine HIV testing of workers in congregate settings (e.g., prisons, shelters, and hospitals) where transmission of TB is most likely.
   C. An effective alternative to a mandatory HIV testing program in the high-risk workplace is a TB screening program that includes PPD screening, voluntary testing for HIV, chest x-rays, and prophylaxis against TB when indicated, augmented by a vigorous educational program. This recommendation does not apply to the average workplace, where the risk is low.
2. Will efforts to protect those with HIV infection from TB require the adoption of restrictive employment practices?
   A. Notions of decency, the moral obligations of employers to employees, and the law—the Occupational Safety and Health Act—require the workplace be made as safe as possible for all employees who may be exposed to TB.
   B. Individuals who are infected with HIV should not be excluded from the workplaces in which they are in danger of contracting TB, especially in facilities where TB transmission is likely to occur.
   C. An extensive education program on TB should be a prominent part of every employee health program, especially in facilities where transmission is likely to occur.
3. What public health policies will be required by the challenge of TB to assure that individuals with the disease are identified and provided with treatment until cured?
   A. In order to enhance the acceptance of TB care, hospitals must provide treatment that is sensitive to the life situation and needs of the patient.
   B. The public health threat posed by TB provides the ethical and legal justifications for extending the period of mandated treatment beyond infectiousness until cure. Society must adopt laws and policies that require and facilitate such treatment.
   C. State and city health agencies must develop a new law that requires treatment until cure and commits the state to creating and implementing appropriate policies and financing programs that will enhance and assure patient compliance.
   D. An evaluation of the post-discharge needs of the patient must include social and psychiatric assessment and a plan to provide appropriate medical and social services, including housing, drug abuse treatment, and mental health care.
   E. The New York City Department of Health and all medical providers should offer social incentives for compliance with regimens of TB treatment until cure.
   F. The New York City Department of Health should encourage, pilot-test, and evaluate programs that employ monetary incentives to encourage completion of therapy.
   G. Directly observed therapy should be required of all TB patients following discharge from a hospital.

Table 14.1, continued

    H. Due process requires that a prompt judicial or administrative hearing with appointed counsel for the poor be convened for any individual who may be confined for noncompliance.

    I. Because of ethical, legal, and pragmatic reasons, those who are confined because of noncompliance should not be compelled to take medication against their will.

Source: N.N. Dubler, R. Bayer, and S. Landesman, "Tuberculosis in the 1990s: Ethical, Legal and Public Policy Issues," in *The Tuberculosis Revival: Individual Rights and Societal Obligations in a Time of AIDS* (New York: United Hospital Fund, 1992). Used with permission.

---

therapy while minimizing restrictions on individual liberty (Iseman, Cohn, & Sbarbaro, 1993).

This concern, among others, occupied the thoughts of a "diverse group of committed, thoughtful scholars, clinicians, administrators, and policymakers" who convened in April of 1992 under the auspices of the United Hospital Fund (1992) to discuss the ethical and legal challenges of TB and to make recommendations for future directions in the containment of this dual epidemic. This group examined three overarching questions that are displayed in Table 14.1. These questions provide readers with an overview of some of the most important ethical and legal concerns associated with the current TB epidemic. Although it is beyond the scope of this book to examine in detail the conclusions of this eminent group, their recommendations are summarized below. Although these recommendations address issues in New York City, they can be extrapolated to the rest of nation. Readers with a special interest in legal and ethical issues related to TB would do well to read the report in its entirety. The report also contains an excellent case study, complete with ethical questions, which might be adapted for classroom teaching and discussion purposes.

All 50 states have laws that give health officers the power to control communicable diseases, including TB (Gostin, 1993). One survey of state laws that apply to the containment of TB concluded that "TB control is largely governed by antiquated laws that predate modern concepts of constitutional law and the need for a flexible range of public health powers" (Gostin, 1993, p.255). Gostin (1993) recommended that future TB control "should focus on effective compliance- enhancing policies, including incentives, social support, education, counseling, drug treatment, housing and employment programs, and better interpersonal communication" (p.260). Finally, noting that "recalcitrance" is an oversimplified concept, Gostin concluded that in employing coercive

TABLE 14.2 Goals for State Tuberculosis Control Programs

States should have systems that incorporate the following guidelines:
1. Ensure the mandatory reporting of each confirmed and suspected case of TB and observe local laws and regulations protecting patient confidentiality;
2. Examine persons for high risk of TB infection and disease, prescribe the appropriate preventive or curative treatment for these persons, and monitor their treatment;
3. Monitor the treatment of patients and require that a treatment plan be devised for all hospitalized patients before they are discharged;
4. Ensure the rapid laboratory examination of specimens and reporting of results to the appropriate health department and requesting clinician;
5. Ensure that TB-infected patients receive treatment until they are cured;
6. Protect the health of the public by isolating and treating persons who have infectious TB and detaining persons who, although not infectious, are unwilling or unable to complete their treatment and are at risk of becoming infectious and acquiring drug-resistant TB;
7. Finance the treatment of indigent patients

---

approaches for a minority of patients that "Health officials should be guided by the principle of the least intrusive alternative necessary to achieve the public health objective" (p. 260).

Another survey, conducted by the Centers for Disease Control and Prevention (CDC) (1993), included TB control officers in all states and the District of Columbia. This survey was aimed at clarifying discrepancies between published recommendations and guidelines for TB control and state TB control laws. The CDC survey questions, which provide insight into a range of ethical and legal issues related to TB control, examined areas such as tuberculosis reporting requirements, populations subject to tuberculosis screening, the nature of tuberculosis control programs, provisions of treatment for persons with TB, and persons restricted from activities and/or employment if infected with TB. This important survey is linked with a set of 25 recommendations for changes in state laws and procedures related to case reporting, provision of treatment, restrictions for persons infected with TB, commitment of persons with infectious TB, treatment facilities, financing of treatment, investigation of TB cases, and TB control officers. The report also contains a detailed table displaying survey findings on a state-by-state basis. The findings from this survey also resulted in the CDC's issuance of seven broad goals for state TB control programs which are displayed in Table 14.2.

CONCLUSION

Nurses need to develop an awareness of the historical and social significance of TB to provide more sensitive care to patients. An understanding of local and state TB laws and the limits of these laws assist nurses in appreciating the social context of TB and the future directions needed to contain the present epidemic. Many state laws that pertain to TB need revision to assure a balance between the individual and public good. The TB epidemic raises important questions about the limits of individual liberty when the health and welfare of others are jeopardized by exposure to those with a communicable disease. Policy makers must resolve many of these questions if public health measures to contain the TB epidemic are to be successfully implemented in ways that are sensitive to the rights of both the few and the many. Inasmuch as nurses are central to interventions aimed at containing the TB epidemic, it behooves nurses in leadership roles to have a thorough grounding in the legal and ethical implications of TB-related policies and practices affecting patients and health care providers.

REFERENCES

American College of Chest Physicians. (1972). Report of the Committee on Tuberculosis: Utilization of general hospitals in the treatment of tuberculosis. *Chest, 61*, 405.

Centers for Disease Control. (1990a). Screening for tuberculosis and tuberculous infection in high risk populations and the use of preventive therapy for tuberculous infection in the United States. *Morbidity and Mortality Weekly Report*, 39(RR–8), 1–12.

Centers for Disease Control. (1990b). Tuberculosis among foreign-born persons entering the United States. *Morbidity and Mortality Weekly Report, 39* (RR–18), 1–21.

Centers for Disease Control. (1992). Prevention and control of tuberculosis in U.S. communities with at-risk minority populations and prevention and control of tuberculosis among homeless persons. *Morbidity and Mortality Weekly Report, 41*(RR–5), 1–23.

Centers for Disease Control. (1993). Tuberculosis control laws: United States, 1993. *Morbidity and Mortality Weekly Report, 42*(RR–15), 1–28.

Gostin, L. (1993). Controlling the resurgent tuberculosis epidemic. *Journal of the American Medical Association, 269* (2), 255–261.

Iseman, M. D., Cohn, D. L., & Sbarbaro, J. A. (1993). Directly observed treatment of tuberculosis. We can't afford not to try it. *New England Journal of Medicine, 328*, 576–578.

Office of Technology Assessment. (1993). The continuing challenge of tuberculosis. Washington, DC: Author.

Rothman, S. (1992). The sanitorium experience: Myths and realities. In United Hospital Fund, *The tuberculosis revival: Individual rights and societal obligations in a time of AIDS* (67–73). NY: United Hospital Fund.

United Hospital Fund. (1992). *The tuberculosis revival: Individual rights and societal obligations in a time of AIDS*. NY: Author.

U.S. Congress. (1992). Tuberculosis, the federal failure: Hearing before the Human Resources and Intergovernmental Relations Subcommittee of the Committee on Government Operations, House of Representatives, April 2, 1992.

U.S. Congress. (1993). The tuberculosis epidemic: Hearing before the Subcommittee on Health and Environment of the Committee on Energy and Commerce, House of Representatives, March 29, 1993.

U.S. Department of Health and Human Services. (1988). *A Strategic Plan for the Elimination of Tuberculosis in the United States*. Washington, DC: Author.

APPENDIX 1

A STRATEGIC PLAN FOR THE ELIMINATION OF TUBERCULOSIS IN THE UNITED STATES

The Advisory Committee for the Elimination of Tuberculosis (ACET) constituted by the U.S. Department of Health and Human Services in 1987 published recommendations in 1989. These recommendations provided a "roadmap" for the effort to eliminate TB in the United States by 2010.

A three-step plan of action is proposed:

Step 1. More effective use of existing prevention and control methods, especially in high-risk populations;

Step 2. The development and evaluation of new technologies for diagnosis, treatment, and prevention; and

Step 3. The rapid assessment and transfer of newly developed technologies into clinical and public health practice.

Current problems cited in the plan include deficiencies in identifying and reporting TB cases and contacts, the failure to fully use prevention interventions, the failure of many patients to complete prescribed therapy, and the failure to adequately assess the effectiveness of community prevention and control programs.

Recommended priorities for action include (1) identifying and screening high-risk population groups within each health jurisdiction and (2) making adequate and appropriate treatment and prophylaxis more available.

The complete report may be found in a special supplement widely distributed to public, private, and voluntary groups to "develop more specific strategies and tactics for implementing the plan" (Centers for Disease Control, 1989, p. 272).

REFERENCE

Centers for Disease Control (1989). A strategic plan for the elimination of tuberculosis in the United States. *Morbidity and Mortality Weekly Report*, 38 (S–3) 1–25.

APPENDIX 2

THE CDC NATIONAL ACTION PLAN TO COMBAT MULTIDRUG-RESISTANT TUBERCULOSIS: A SYNOPSIS

SURVEILLANCE AND EPIDEMIOLOGY
Determine the magnitude and nature of the problem of MDR-TB.

Problem 1: National surveillance systems are inadequate to accurately determine the frequency and patterns of drug-resistant TB.

Objective 1: Develop nationwide surveillance systems for determining the drug susceptibility patterns of persons with active TB.

Problem 2: Hospitals, correctional facilities, and other institutional settings have been the focus of outbreaks of MDR-TB. The extent of MDR-TB transmission in the community has not been well studied. Epidemiologic studies and surveillance data are needed to assess the risk of infection and disease and factors promoting TB transmission in institutional settings, as well as the extent of community transmission.

Objective 2: Conduct epidemiologic investigations and studies to better define the scope and magnitude of the problem, to identify risk factors for transmission of TB in special settings, and to define the extent of MDR-TB transmission in the community.

Problem 3: Certain subgroups of the population, including workers and clients of some service occupations, are at increased risk of TB. Data are needed to assess the risks and patterns of *M. tuberculosis* infection and active TB (both MDR-TB and drug-sensitive TB) among workers and others in settings where there is a risk of TB transmission.

Objective 3: Determine the patterns of TB disease and infection among workers and others in settings where there is a risk of TB transmission and characterize current programs for TB infection screening and infection control in these settings.

Problem 4: Persons with HIV infection have been the focus of recent MDR-TB outbreaks; however, the impact of HIV infection on TB trends has not been well characterized. Information is needed to assess the impact of HIV infection on recent trends in TB disease and infection, including MDR-TB, in the United States.

Objective 4a: Characterize the HIV infection status of persons with TB and forecast the effect of HIV on future TB trends.

Objective 4b: Study drug-susceptibility patterns, treatment, and risk factors for TB among HIV infected persons and perform surveillance of skin-test reactivity, anergy testing, and use of preventive therapy for persons with HIV infection.

LABORATORY DIAGNOSIS
Make the laboratory diagnosis of MDR-TB more rapid, sensitive, and reliable.

Problem 5: The most rapid currently available laboratory technologies to identify MDR-TB are not in widespread use in state and local health department laboratories.

Objective 5: Increase the awareness and understanding of MDR-TB in the laboratory community and upgrade the mycobacteriology capacity of state and local public health laboratories.

Problem 6:   As the outbreak spreads to more geographic areas, current laboratory capacity to track and characterize the epidemic of MDR-TB may not be adequate.

Objective 6:   Enhance laboratory capacity to support outbreak investigations and special studies of MDR-TB.

Problem 7:   Approximately 700,000 aliens[1] apply for permanent resident status annually in the United States. Under provisions of the Immigration and Nationality Act, each of these persons must receive a medical examination that includes an examination for TB. The quality of laboratories used by examining physicians abroad may not be adequate to perform sputum smear examinations to identify infectious TB or to perform drug-susceptibility tests.

Objective 7:   Evaluate the ability of these overseas screening laboratories to detect acid-fast bacilli, identify *M. tuberculosis*, and carry out drug-susceptibility tests; enhance their capability as needed.

PATIENT MANAGEMENT

Prevent patients with drug-susceptible TB from developing drug-resistant disease. Effectively manage patients who have developed drug-resistant disease.

Problem 8:   TB treatment must be given for a minimum of 6 to 9 months. If TB patients do not complete therapy, they may not be cured, and if they take medications incorrectly, the organisms may become drug resistant. Therefore, TB patients need some degree of supervision to ensure compliance with and completion of therapy.

Objective 8:   Provide guidance regarding a step-wise approach to assure completion of therapy for all TB patients, with particular emphasis on implementation of directly observed therapy (DOT).

Problem 9:   Approximately 700,000 aliens apply for immigrant visas abroad annually. Many of these applicants live in countries that have a high incidence of MDR-TB because of inadequate programs for managing and treating persons with TB.

---

[1] The term "alien" is defined in the U. S. Immmigration and Nationality Act as any person who is not a citizen or national of the United States.

Objective 9: To decrease the likelihood of introduction of MDR-TB to the United States, evaluate the feasibility of establishing DOT programs in four or five of the countries from which a high volume of immigration originates and which have a high incidence of TB.

Problem 10: Few inpatient facilities are available for long-term treatment of patients with complicated TB cases, particularly those with MDR-TB, and many areas do not have a method of paying for these services.

Objective 10: Explore varying options for long-term institutionalization of TB patients, including patients with MDR-TB, and assist health departments in securing Medicare, Medicaid, and other funds for financing institutional care.

Problem 11: Many TB patients do not have health insurance. Local health department budgets have difficulty providing adequate services to all who need them. Resultant breaks in the continuity of care may lead to the development of drug-resistant disease.

Objective 11: Find means to pay for outpatient services to persons who do not have third-party coverage.

Problem 12: TB patients, particularly those with MDR-TB, often require specialized services that are difficult to provide in all acute-care hospitals and outpatient clinics.

Objective 12: Evaluate the feasibility of developing specialized inpatient and outpatient TB treatment units and regional inpatient treatment centers.

Problem 13: Drugs needed to treat TB, particularly MDR-TB, are often unavailable, and some of them are expensive, which may be an obstacle to effective treatment.

Objective 13: CDC, Food and Drug Administration (FDA), pharmaceutical manufacturers, and others will work together to assure an ongoing supply of currently licensed antituberculosis drugs at an acceptable cost.

Problem 14: Laws, regulations, and/or procedures for the quarantine, detention, reporting, and treatment of patients may be out of date or inadequate as the epidemiology of TB continues to evolve.

Objective 14: Develop guidelines and recommendations that address the legal issues of TB control.

Problem 15:   Homeless TB patients are often not able to complete TB therapy because of lack of stable housing and need for other social services; as a result, drug-resistant disease may develop.

Objective 15:   TB patients who are homeless, have unstable living arrangements, or lack essential social services will have access to housing for the duration of their TB treatment and will receive assistance with social services.

Problem 16:   TB among migrant and seasonal farmworkers may be undiagnosed and inadequately treated because of lack of stable housing, the unique work situation, and geographic mobility; as a result, drug-resistant disease may develop.

Objective 16:   Coordinate public health systems so that migrant and seasonal farmworkers have access to diagnosis and treatment.

Problem 17:   TB patients who have substance abuse problems are likely to be noncompliant with TB therapy and may develop drug-resistant disease as a result.

Objective 17a: Improve patient compliance with antituberculosis regimens among substance abusers in drug-abuse treatment centers.

Objective 17b: Improve patient compliance with antituberculosis regimens among substance abusers not in drug-abuse treatment programs.

Problem 18:   Approximately 700,000 aliens apply for permanent resident status annually. A large percentage of these applicants come from countries where TB (including MDR-TB) is common. Under provisions of the Immigration and Nationality Act, many aliens with active TB are admitted to the United States with a waiver of excludability. When such persons arrive at a U.S. Port of Entry (POE), CDC staff notifies state and local health authorities at the final destination. However, CDC does not have staff at all major POEs and must rely on the Immigration and Naturalization Service staff to provide copies of the aliens' medical documentation so that health authorities can be notified. Consequently, notification on some aliens arriving with TB is missed, with resultant breaks in continuity of care and possibility of drug-resistant disease.

Objective 18:   Improve the process of notifying state and local health departments about aliens arriving with TB.

SCREENING AND PREVENTIVE THERAPY
Identify persons who are infected with or at risk of developing MDR-TB and prevent them from developing clinically active TB.

Problem 19:   A standard approach to the evaluation and management of persons exposed to MDR-TB is lacking.

Objective 19:   Develop and publish an approach to the evaluation and management of persons exposed to MDR-TB.

Problem 20:   Many persons in populations at high risk for TB may also be at risk for noncompliance with therapy if active TB develops; as a result, drug-resistant TB may develop.

Objective 20:   Implement screening and preventive therapy programs, including supervised preventive therapy, among populations at high risk for both TB and noncompliance.

INFECTION CONTROL
Minimize the risk of transmission of MDR- TB to patients, workers, and others in institutional settings.

Problem 21:   Various infection control strategies are available to prevent TB transmission in institutional settings. These strategies are not consistently implemented, and their effectiveness and feasibility are not well characterized.

Objective 21:   Assess the effectiveness and feasibility of various infection control strategies in institutional settings (e.g., health-care facilities, substance abuse clinics, residential treatment centers, shelters for the homeless, correctional facilities) and ensure that appropriate procedures are implemented through educational and regulatory approaches.

Problem 22:   Tuberculin skin testing of workers in settings where there is a risk of TB transmission is very important. Skin testing identifies workers who are infected with *M. tuberculosis* and need to be evaluated for active TB and for preventive therapy. It also serves as an indicator of the effectiveness of infection control practices. However, tuberculin skin-testing programs are not consistently implemented.

Objective 22:   Ensure that adequate tuberculin skin-testing pro-
                grams for workers are in place in settings where
                there is a substantial risk of TB transmission.

OUTBREAK CONTROL
Control Outbreaks of MDR-TB

Problem 23:   The control of MDR-TB outbreaks is costly and
                complex, requiring close collaboration among lo-
                cal, state, and federal health officials and others
                (e.g., hospital officials, correctional facility offi-
                cials, technical consultants.)
Objective 23:   Facilitate collaboration of various officials and or-
                ganizations in controlling MDR-TB outbreaks.

PROGRAM EVALUATION
Evaluate TB control programs to be sure they are effective in managing
patients and preventing the development of MDR-TB.

Problem 24:   Some TB control programs may not be effective
                in managing TB patients, which may allow drug-
                resistant disease to develop. There is a need for
                assessing the quality of TB control (including
                health department infrastructure, facilities, and
                priorities).
Objective 24:   CDC, in conjunction with other agencies (e.g., the
                American Lung Association [ALA], other mem-
                bers of the National Coalition for Elimination of
                TB), will assist state and local health departments
                in assessing the adequacy of their TB control pro-
                grams.
Problem 25:   Poor compliance with prescribed treatment pro-
                motes the development of drug-resistant strains of
                M. tuberculosis, which may lead to outbreaks of
                MDR-TB. Programs do not currently collect and
                analyze data on treatment outcomes that would
                identify populations at high risk for treatment
                failure.
Objective 25:   Assess program performance by collecting infor-
                mation on treatment outcomes of TB patients on
                an individual case basis, which will allow more
                effective targeting of resources.

INFORMATION DISSEMINATION/TRAINING AND EDUCATION
Effectively disseminate information about MDR-TB and its prevention and control.

Problem 26:   Expertise regarding treatment of TB, especially MDR-TB, is lacking in many parts of the United States.

Objective 26:   Develop a cadre of health-care professionals with expertise in the management of TB, including MDR-TB.

Problem 27:   Nosocomial transmission of TB to health-care workers and patients is occurring. Such transmission is preventable if recommended infection control practices are implemented.

Objective 27:   Disseminate information on the prevention of TB transmission to individuals and in facilities that provide services to persons who already have TB or who are at high risk for it.

Problem 28:   A critical need exists for trained researchers to develop new diagnostic assays, therapeutic agents, and vaccines to meet present and future TB public health needs.

Objective 28:   Train adequate numbers of researchers to respond effectively to TB research needs.

Problem 29:   Mycobacteriology laboratory personnel may not be familiar with state-of-the-art TB diagnostic technologies and reporting practices.

Objective 29:   Provide training and evaluation of clinical mycobacteriology laboratory personnel in new diagnostic techniques for TB.

Problem 30:   Strategies for training and delivering TB information and education to health professionals and others have been inadequate.

Objective 30:   Develop an integrated system for professional information and communication on TB.

RESEARCH
Perform research to identify better methods for combatting MDR-TB.

Problem 31:   Research on TB needs to be conducted and promoted by a variety of agencies, including CDC, NIH, FDA, and others. Coordination of research efforts among these agencies will be important in ensuring that critical knowledge gaps are addressed effectively.

Objective 31: Develop a mechanism for coordinating TB research activities among the various agencies involved.

Problem 32: There is a critical lack of knowledge about the basic characteristics of *M. tuberculosis* (e.g., growth, physiology, biochemistry, genetics, and molecular biology). This knowledge gap is a barrier to the development of new treatment and control modalities.

Objective 32: Provide increased support for basic research on the biology of *M. tuberculosis* and the host responses to infection.

Problem 33: Existing diagnostic methods to identify persons with drug-resistant TB are very slow, impeding treatment and control efforts.

Objective 33: Develop and evaluate new technology to rapidly and reliably diagnose cases of TB and identify patterns of drug susceptibility.

Problem 34: Existing methods for identifying latent TB infection, especially among persons who are immunosuppressed, lack sensitivity and specificity.

Objective 34: Develop and evaluate new technologies to rapidly and reliably identify latent tuberculous infection among both immunocompetent and immunosuppressed persons.

Problem 35: Currently available drugs are not sufficiently effective in treating MDR-TB. The duration of therapy required to treat TB with currently available drugs leads to noncompliance with therapy and development of drug-resistance disease.

Objective 35: Encourage the development and evaluation of new drugs and modalities to treat and prevent MDR-TB, as well as to reduce the duration of therapy required to cure drug-susceptible TB.

Problem 36: Currently available vaccines against TB are not reliably effective in preventing acquisition of TB.

Objective 36: Develop and evaluate new and improved vaccines to prevent infection and disease with *M. tuberculosis*.

Problem 37: The efficacy of various technologies for preventing TB transmission (e.g., general and local ventilation, UVGI, and personal protective equipment) has not been adequately evaluated.

Objective 37:   Conduct basic and applied research on the efficacy and role of various control methods for preventing transmission of TB.

Problem 38:   Poor patient compliance leads to development of MDR-TB. Compliance is influenced by patient characteristics; characteristics of the health-care environment, including operational factors and compliance-enhancing intervention; and communication between patient and providers, including the quality of interpersonal communication and use of educational materials for transfer of information about the nature of the disease and treatment.

Objective 38:   Identify ways to improve compliance with therapy through behavioral research.

Source: Centers for Disease Control and Prevention. (1992). National action plan to combat multidrug-resistant tuberculosis. *Morbidity and Mortality Weekly Report*, *41(No. RR-11)*, 1–48.

APPENDIX 3

SOURCES FOR EDUCATIONAL MATERIALS FOR PATIENTS AND HEALTH-CARE WORKERS

In addition to the material listed below, organizations and periodicals that specialize in HIV/AIDS content may also have information on TB as it relates to HIV disease.

Organizations
American Academy of Pediatrics, Committee on Infectious Diseases
141 N.W. Point Blvd
Elk Grove Village, IL 60007

American Lung Association
1740 Broadway
New York, NY 10019-4374
(212) 315-8700
    Medical Section:
    American Thoracic Society (ATS)
    1740 Broadway
    New York, NY 10019-4375
    Publishes *ATS News*; has various Assemblies under the ATS, including the Nursing Assembly.
    The ALA has chapters and branches in areas across the country.

American Public Health Association
1015 Fifteenth St., NW
Washington, DC 20005

Association for Practitioners in Infection Control
505 East Hawley St.
Mundelein, IL 60060

Centers for Disease Control and Prevention (CDC)
National Center for Prevention Services
Division of Tuberculosis Elimination
Atlanta, Georgia, 30333
(404) 639-2508
The CDC have many available booklets, slides, and posters on TB.

Infectious Diseases Society of America
c/o Vincent T. Andriole, M.D.
Yale University School of Medicine
333 Cedar St., 201 LCI
New Haven, CT 06510-8056

Association for Professionals in Infection Control and Epidemiology, Inc.
1016 Sixteenth St, NW, 6th floor
Washington, DC, 20036
(202) 296-2742

International Union Against Tuberculosis and Lung Diseases
68 Boulevard Saint Michel
75006, Paris, France

Respiratory Nursing Society
5700 Old Orchard Rd, First Floor
Skokie, IL 60077-1057
(708) 966-8673
Publishes *Perspectives in Respiratory Nursing*

World Health Organization
Tuberculosis Programme
Geneva, Switzerland

Selected Publications and Statements
In addition to this list, most state health departments and affiliates of the American Lung Association offer professional and/or lay information relating to TB,including tuberculin skin testing, medication information,and other literature. Many organizations offer material in other languages such as Spanish, Vietnamese, Polish, Russian, Laotian, Korean,

French, Greek, Creole, Farsi, Chinese, Japanese, Cambodian, and Tagalog.

American Hospital Association, Technical Panel on Infections.(1994). *Tuberculosis control in hospitals. A special briefing.* Chicago, Illinois, American Hospital Association, AHA Catalog No. 094692.

American Lung Association. (1993). *Tuberculosis education resource guide*, New York, NY, American Lung Association. This guide lists audiovisual materials on TB for patients and professionals.

American Lung Association of South Carolina. (1989). *Tuberculosis control: enablers and incentives.* Columbia, South Carolina.

American Nurses Association. (1993). *Position statement on tuberculosis and public health nursing.* Washington, DC.

American Thoracic Society. (1992). Control of tuberculosis in the United States. *American Review of Respiratory Disease, 146,* 1623-1633.

American Thoracic Society. (1990). Diagnostic standards and classification of tuberculosis. *American Review of Respiratory Disease, 142,* 725-735.

Centers for Disease Control and Prevention. *Core curriculum on tuberculosis.* Atlanta, GA, Centers for Disease Control and Prevention, 1994.

Centers for Disease Control and Prevention. *Control of tuberculosis in correctional facilities. A guide for health care workers,*(DHHS Publication No. 632-867). Washington, D.C. U.S. Government Printing Office.

Centers for Disease Control and Prevention. *TB facts for health care workers. Think TB.* Revised 1993.

National Institute of Allergy and Infectious Disease, NIH. (1992). *Backgrounder: Tuberculosis.*

National Institute for Occupational Safety and Health. (1993). *NIOSH recommended guidelines of personal respiratory protection of workers in health care facilities potentially exposed to tuberculosis.* Atlanta, Centers for Disease Control and Prevention.

Office of Technology Assessment. 1993. *The continuing challenge of tuberculosis.* Washington, D.C., Author.

Snider, D.E. & Hutton, M.D. *Improving patient compliance in tuberculosis treatment programs.* Atlanta, Georgia, Centers for Disease Control, 1989.

Tuberculosis and HIV disease. A report of the Special Initiative on AIDS of the American Public Health Association, November, 1992.

U.S. Congress. (1993). *The tuberculosis epidemic: Hearing before the Subcommittee on Health and Environment of the Committee on Energy and Commerce, House of Representatives*, March 29, 1993. Available from U.S. Government Printing Office.

Other information from Centers for Disease Control and Prevention:
Tuberculosis: Get the facts!
Tuberculosis facts—Exposure to TB.
Tuberculosis facts—The TB skin test.
Tuberculosis facts—TB and HIV
Tuberculosis facts—You can prevent TB
Tuberculosis facts—TB can be cured
(Spanish versions of these are available.)

Screening for tuberculosis: Administering and reading the Mantoux Test. Videotape 0260-CPS.

Selected issues of Recommendations and Reports, and Surveillance Summaries that are published as special issues of the *Morbidity and Mortality Weekly Report* are specific to TB. Many of these are referenced in this book within the appropriate chapter.

This is not an exhaustive list. Other materials are available from CDC.

Selected Journals and Serials Frequently Featuring Articles on TB
Advances in Pediatric Infectious Diseases
American Journal of Infection Control
American Journal of Public Health
American Journal of Respiratory and Critical Care Medicine (formerly
    American Review of Respiratory Disease)
Chest
Clinical Infectious Diseases
Clinics in Chest Medicine
Current Pulmonology
European Respiratory Journal
Indian Journal of Tuberculosis
Infection Control and Hospital Epidemiology
Journal of Infectious Diseases
Journal of Respiratory Diseases
Lung and Respiration
Lung Biology in Health and Disease

Morbidity and Mortality Weekly Reports
Pediatric Infectious Disease Journal
Respiration
Respiratory Care
Respiratory Medicine
Thorax
Tubercle and Lung Disease
Year Book of Pulmonary Medicine

GLOSSARY

Acid-fast bacilli (AFB)—Bacteria that retain certain stains after being washed with acid alcohol. The mycobacteria, including *Mycobacterium tuberculosis*, have this property.

Acquired drug resistance—Resistance to one or more drugs that develops after the person is on drug therapy

Adherence—Also called compliance. Refers to a person complying with all aspects of their treatment regimen.

Anergy—The inability of a person to react to skin-test antigens because of defects in delayed hypersensitivity. The person may still have tuberculous infection but not be able to mount an immune response to the test antigen.

Bacteriocidal—Agent that can kill bacteria

Bacteriostatic—Agent that prevents bacterial growth but does not kill bacteria

BCG vaccine—Bacille de Calmette Guérin vaccine that is an attenuated strain of *Mycobacterium bovis* and is used to protect against tuberculosis

Booster phenomenon—The booster effect or recall phenomenon is based on the waning of delayed-type hypersensitivity (DTH) over time and its recall by a subsequent tuberculin skin test

Caseous—A type of tissue necrosis that has a cheeselike consistency

Cell-mediated immunity—A type of immune reactivity in which T lymphocytes participate

Contact—A person who has shared the same air with a person with infectious TB. It usually means that there is a probability of transmission of TB occurring.

Culture—Growing microorganisms in the laboratory for their identification

Delayed hypersensitivity—A type of cell-mediated immune response that occurs when T cells encounter their specific antigen and lymphokines are released

Directly observed therapy (DOT)—Treatment in which each medication dose is taken under the supervision of a health care worker or trained person

Droplet nuclei—Microscopic particles produced when a person coughs, sneezes, sings, or shouts. These droplets (1–5 microns in diameter) can carry *M. tuberculosis*, and can remain in the room air.

Drug-resistant TB—TB that is not susceptible or is resistant to one or more anti-TB medications

Exogenous reinfection—Tuberculosis caused by an external source of *M. tuberculosis* in someone who had a previous tuberculous infection

Endogenous reactivation—Reactivation of dormant foci of *M. tuberculosis* that were in the body from a previous infection

Ghon complex—A parenchymal lung lesion resulting from healing of the primary inflammation due to tuberculous infection

HEPA filter—A high efficiency particulate air filter that removes almost all air particles greater than 0.3 microns in diameter and is used in TB control

Induration—The area of firmness or swelling that surrounds the tuberculin injection site and is read in millimeters as the reaction to the Mantoux test

In vivo—In the living organism

In vitro—In the laboratory or test tube

Koch, Robert—Scientist who discovered the bacterium causing TB

Mantoux test—A type of tuberculin skin test in which the test material is introduced intradermally

Miliary tuberculosis—A type of TB that is hematogenous or generalized; so-called because the seeding causes lesions that resembles millet seeds.

Multidrug-resistant TB—Case of tuberculosis caused by a strain of *Mycobacterium tuberculosis* resistant to two or more antituberculosis drugs

Mycobacterium tuberculosis—The microorganism causing tuberculosis

Old tuberculin (OT)—A filtrate prepared from sterilized concentrates of *M. tuberculosis* used in tuberculin testing with multiple puncture devices

Positive PPD Reaction—Reaction to tuberculin skin testing with PPD (see below) that suggests the person has been infected wtih tubercule bacilli

Primary drug resistance—Infection with an organism that has spontaneously mutated to become resistant to the drug

Primary tuberculosis—Refers to TB that occurs in a person not previously infected with *M. tuberculosis*

Purified protein derivative (PPD)—A precipitate prepared from OT that is used with either multiple puncture testing devices or intradermally via the Mantoux test

Ranke Complex—A combination of the Ghon lesion and calcification in a hilar node in the lung

Source case—A person who has transmitted TB to another

Tine test—A type of multiple puncture tuberculin skin test

Tubercle bacilli—A collective term to refer to organisms in the *Mycobacterium tuberculosis* complex or to *M. tuberculosis*

Tuberculosis (TB)—A chronic bacterial infection due to *Mycobacterium tuberculosis*, characterized pathologically by the formation of granulomas. The most common site is the lung (pulmonary TB), but other organs may be involved (extrapulmonary TB).

White plague—A name given to tuberculosis

Virulence—The ability of a micro-organism to produce disease

INDEX

CHESTER COLLEGE LIBRARY

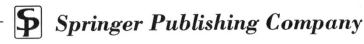 *Springer Publishing Company*

DELIVERING HEALTH CARE TO HOMELESS PERSONS

The Diagnosis and Management of Medical and Mental Health Conditions

David Wood, MD, MPH, Editor

Outlines innovative approaches to providing health care to America's homeless population children as well as adults. The perspective is patient-oriented, emphasizing on-site and community-based care. Encompasses case management from medical, social, and psychological viewpoints.

"...fills a growing need for a reference on the spectrum of health problems of the homeless in America."

—Nurse Practitioner

Contents:

Named a "Best Book of 1992" by Nurse Practitioner

1992   304pp   0-8261-7780-8   hard $38.95 (outside US $44.50)

536 Broadway, New York, NY 10012-3955 • (212) 431-4370 • Fax (212) 941-7842

$ *Springer Publishing Company*

THE HEALTH OF POPULATIONS
An Introduction, 2nd Edition

Andrew C. Harper, MPH, DrPH, and
Laurie Lambert, B Phys Ed

This text provides a framework for understanding the determinants of a community's health. The authors discuss the role services and other measures play in improving the physical and mental well-being of a population. The new edition provides updated information, numbers, examples, and references. There is also new material on the historical development of population health.

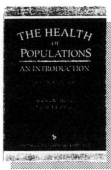

"...*a readable introductory text in epidemiology that conveys an overview of the field without the pain associated by most students with this topic.*"

—Journal of Health Administration Education

Partial Contents:

I. A Framework for a Population Perspective • The Problem: A General Perspective on Health • The Problem: The Health of Specific Populations • Risks 1: History and Concepts • Risks 2: Causes of Disease • Risks 3: Selected Diseases and Their Causes • Solutions 1: Reducing the Risk of Disease • Solutions 2: The Search for Effective Therapy • Solutions 3: The Role of the Health Care System • Population Health in Perspective

1993   296pp   0-8261-5511-1   softcover

536 Broadway, New York, NY 10012-3955 • (212) 431-4370 • Fax (212) 941-7842

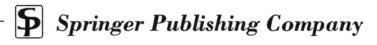
Springer Publishing Company

THE PERSON WITH AIDS
Nursing Perspectives, 2nd Edition

Jerry D. Durham, RN, PhD, FAAN
and **Felissa L. Cohen**, RN, PhD, FAAN, Editors

Completely revised and expanded edition of the first comprehensive resource for AIDS for nurses, covers all aspects of working with people with HIV / AIDS. Includes epidemiological and psychosocial aspects, prevention, home care, acute care, discharge planning as well as ethical and legal issues. The clinical chapters provide hands-on information and care procedures/plans.

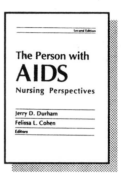

The Person with
AIDS
Nursing Perspectives

Jerry D. Durham
Felissa L. Cohen
Editors

About the First Edition

"...thorough and scholarly...offers a cutting-edge discussion of AIDS"

—American Journal of Nursing

Contents:

The Etiology and Epidemiology of HIV Infection and AIDS • Immune Mechanisms in AIDS • HIV Testing and Counseling • Preventing Clinical Spectrum of HIV Infection and Its Treatments • Nursing Care of Acutely Ill Persons with AIDS • Creating and Managing a Therapeutic Environment: Institutional Settings • Discharge Planning • Sustaining Care of Persons with AIDS • The Impact of HIV Infection on Women • The Child with HIV Infection • Future Treatments, Alternate Therapies and Vaccine Development • Ethical/Legal Dimensions of AIDS • AIDS: The Politics of a Pandemic • Appendices

Nurse's Book Society Selection. Translated into Spanish.

1991   448pp   0-8261-5631-2 hardcover

536 Broadway, New York, NY 10012-3955 • (212) 431-4370 • Fax (212) 941-7842

$\boxed{\text{SP}}$ Springer Publishing Company

WOMEN, CHILDREN, AND HIV / AIDS

Felissa L. Cohen, RN, PhD, FAAN,
and **Jerry D. Durham**, RN, PhD, FAAN, Editors

"This timely text provides nurses with cutting-edge information on HIV disease and explores the various issues specific to these populations. The context is accurate and comprehensive..."

—American Journal of Nursing

"Women, Children, and HIV / AIDS is a landmark publication...Compiled by a dedicated cadre of nursing authorities, it takes a totally realistic, deep look at current conditions and expectations, and blends it with forward-looking clinical advise for helping women and children living with HIV / AIDS."

—Nurse's Book Society

Contents:

1993   328pp   0-8261-7880-4   hardcover

536 Broadway, New York, NY 10012-3955 • (212) 431-4370 • Fax (212) 941-7842